PTCB Exam

Prep

2023-2024

Study Guide with 270 Practice
Questions and Answer Explanations
for the Pharmacy Technician
Certification Board Test

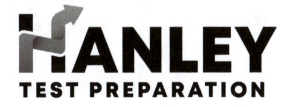

Contents

Introduction

There are no secrets to success. It is the result of preparation, hard work, and learning from failure.

— Colin Powell

Naturally, when you prepare to take any type of board exam, your stress levels tend to increase dramatically. However, some types of board exams can be a bit more mentally strenuous than others. An example of this is the Pharmacy Technician Certification Board (PTCB) exam. Also, for many, there is a degree of uncertainty about how to prepare for these board exams.

Let's provide some context! If we were to look at the cumulative pass rate of the PTCB exam over the past seven years, it is only 59%. Now, this can be a fear-inducing statistic to read, and we completely understand your apprehension. The best way to make sure you are as prepared as possible is by not sugar-coating the facts. Yes, the exam is hard, but the more you know, the better you are able to prepare yourself.

If we were to take a bird's-eye view of the PTCB pass rate in 2020, it was 70%, which is much higher than the previous years. But we all await the pass rate of the 2021 class, seeing as the pass rate has yet to be published. But let's place the 2020 pass rate into perspective. Amongst other years where the results ranged between 57% and 58%, was there any specific reason for such a large disparity? Some will say COVID-19 resulted in more students studying instead of socializing, and others will say they used specific guides. Either way, it is a marked increase!

Between 2007 and 2013, pass rates started to rise from 70% to 76% before tumbling down to 57% in 2014. For the next five years, there was an exam pass rate of approximately 57% until our most recent 2020's result. So, was the 2020 pass rate the beginning of much higher pass rates? Only time will tell, especially as we wait for the results of the 2021 exam.

Among many other questions students have about the exam, one of the most common is, "How many people will be able to pass the PTCB on their first try?" For many, passing the first time is more about saving time in extra studying and the money needed to pay to write the board exam. You can imagine how much money it can cost if you need to pay for each PTCB exam you need to retake. Another little pothole is that those who do not pass their initial attempt will need to wait 60 days before they can try the exam again. Fast-track this to some applicants who fail the exam on their third attempt; the timeframe you need to wait before trying for the fourth time is six months.

But, although this sounds scary, knowing what to study, how to study effectively, as well as making sure that you do PTCB practice tests will drastically improve your chances of passing the exam. This entire process also means that you need to be completely honest with yourself regarding any strengths and weaknesses you may have in terms of understanding specific categories of content. The parts you struggle more with may need more time, whereas those you are comfortable with may not necessarily need to be studied as intensely.

We understand how you are feeling. The anxiety that comes with writing the board exam, coupled with the stress of needing to plot how long in advance you need to study, can be crippling. But, take this book as your personalized test preparation program, where it is guaranteed that you will be prepared for your next PTCB exam attempt. This handbook is a lot more than just a study guide. It is a practical approach toward giving you an extra advantage over the rest of those taking the exam. With that, there are a bunch of different ways you will be able to benefit from using this preparation handbook. A few of them are as follows:

- Improved memorization: When concepts are explained, the methods present within this handbook are of such an art that they are easy to digest, making memorization that much easier.
- Improved confidence: When you run blindly into an exam, not knowing if you have covered all the content, especially if all your notes were all over the place, you will lose confidence in your academic abilities. With this exam prep handbook, you will be that much more confident to take on the challenge!
- Less anxiety: It is well known that taking any kind of test or exam can be a stressful situation. As you use this handbook and work through all the material offered, you will find yourself more prepared and with less anxiety.
- Time management: If you are either a daytime studier or a night owl, and you don't know how to study given strict limits, then handbooks like this are perfect for you! Not only will you be able to jump into all the required content, but the practice tests in this guide will also encourage you to understand your pacing and where you should allocate your stamina!
- Accessibility to a study guide and full-length practice tests that mimic the actual exam: If you know what to expect in an exam, you are able to properly prepare yourself for what lies ahead. You can do it, and this is the perfect guide to make sure you are successful!

As you jump into taking the PTCB exam, you should start becoming excited at the prospect of becoming a certified pharmacy technician. There are a myriad of benefits you can expect when deciding to take the PTCB exam. For example, those with a PTCB certification will undoubtedly earn higher salaries than pharmacy technicians who do not have this certification. A few further benefits include:

- Those pharmacy professionals who have a PTCB certification will have a higher caliber to uphold patient safety, as well as be more competent in the services provided at a pharmacy.
- Those with a PTCB certification will most likely be given more responsibility at the pharmacy whilst being a few steps ahead of those who don't have the certification. This becomes important when your aim is to move up in the ranks of the pharmacy.

- Apart from already standing out from all your colleagues, the certification will even allow you the ability to comply with legal requirements and practice in respective states that require the PTCB certification for possible employment.
- Along with the ability to practice, the PTCB certification is a reflection of your dedication to gaining knowledge in your field. It is a symbol of achievement, one you should be proud of!

Grasping all of these benefits should be more than enough motivation to really gun toward obtaining your PTCB qualification. Now although you are going to be tested in four categories, namely medications, federal requirements, patient safety and quality assurance, and order entry and processing, you need to be ready to answer these in a Multiple-Choice Question (MCQ) format. We must caution you, though, MCQ exams aren't easy because the answer is already there. They are notoriously difficult because they will use similar answers to confuse you. But, we believe in your ability to use the resources in this guide to really overcome all obstacles and pass the PTCB certification exam with flying colors!

Your journey toward becoming PTCB certified has begun, and we are so excited to be on this journey with you!

Chapter One: The PTCB Exam

The contents of this chapter are going to focus on what the PTCB examination actually is, what it entails, what you need to study, a few important study habits, and all of the eligibility requirements to be allowed access to the exam. But, before we get into all of the science and legal-based content, we need to discuss the PTCB a bit more.

Have you ever wondered how life would be on the other side of the pharmacy counter? A life where a pharmacy technician works in environments that are clean and bright. A pharmacy technician plays an important role in the public's everyday functioning. They act by linking a prescription to a specific individual, ensuring they are given the medication necessary to cure disease, manage chronic conditions, and ultimately live happier and healthier lives. So, what is stopping you from becoming one of these pharmacy technicians? Well . . . all that stands in your way is the PTCB exam.

Is the PTCB Required?

Now you may be asking whether becoming a pharmacy technician means you need to pass this exam. In most cases, this is true. The reason we say in "most cases" is because depending on what state you want to practice in, most states will require you to hold some sort of national certification or form of license as of 2020. Now although there is a national certification exam that the National Healthcare Association (NHA) offers, the PTCB is the one that is most commonly recognized across most states in the USA.

The PTCB is a qualification that is very important to obtain. That is if you see yourself practicing in the USA and have the need to progress personally and professionally within the pharmacist technician domain. Now even though employers will most likely look to see if you have passed your PTCB, having this certification is a requirement for pharmacy technicians to legally handle medications, vaccinations, and prescriptions.

What Can You Expect When Taking the PTCB Exam?

As mentioned previously, the PTCB exam consists of 90 MCQs. However, only 80 of these questions are actually scored, giving you an overall score out of 80 marks. Now, what about the other 10? Well, they just don't count. But they are also scattered throughout your exam, meaning you won't know which question will count or not. This means you really need to remain focused on each and every question throughout the exam. The length of the exam is 1 hour and 50 minutes. This means you will have approximately 1 minute and 22 seconds to answer each question.

Now let's chat about mental preparedness for the exam. You can expect to feel a bit stressed out as the date of the exam draws closer. This is completely normal. In fact, it is scientifically proven that a bit of nerve before an exam can actually help you perform better than you thought was possible. That is if you are able to contain your stress and anxiety! But, knowing that you have studied hard should bring a sense of calmness to your frazzled brain. You've worked hard, and by reminding yourself of that, you will be able to calm down and ace the exam!

What Topics Are Covered in the Exam?

You have already been acquainted with the four different knowledge domains that will be covered in your exam. But, within each of these domains exists subdomains from which your questions will be derived. Expect questions to come from the following subdomains:

- Clinical pharmacology for technicians
- All about pharmacy law and regulations
- Compounding in both a sterile and non-sterile fashion
- Medication safety
- Quality assurance within the pharmacy
- The order and fill process of medication
- Inventory management within the pharmacy
- Billing and reimbursement associated with the pharmacy
- How to use and apply information systems within the pharmacy

Now, this may seem like a lot of content, and it is, but what is great is the inter-connectedness of all these subdomains of knowledge. The knowledge you learn and study will be applicable across more than one knowledge domain. With this in mind, studying hard means you won't spend as much time as you would've constantly revising the same topic. Study hard and finish the content faster—that is how you should approach this.

An In-Depth Content Outline

Now although four main knowledge domains are going to be tested during your PTCB exam, that does not necessarily mean that their weighting in terms of how often questions in those domains appear, will be equal. But this makes sense. After all, as a pharmacy technician, you are going to be dealing with a lot of different medications, which is why the "medications" domain accounts for 40% of the entire exam.

Although important, the "federal requirements" portion does not have as much content that needs to be studied. This is why it only consists of 12.5% of the exam. As a pharmacy technician, you will always need to ensure the safety of your patients, making sure that the medication you provide them with is of the highest quality possible. Thus, the "patient safety and quality assurance" section accounts for 26.25% of the exam. Finally, ensuring that you replenish stock, as well as knowing how to order and process received and issued medications, is important. It is for this reason that the "order entry and processing" domain weighs 21.25% of the exam.

The Medications Domain

As you delve into the medications knowledge domain, you will be required to have an in-depth understanding of the following concepts:

- The classifications of different medications.
- A medication's brand name, generic name, and active ingredient.
- What the term "therapeutic equivalence" means, and how it is applied within the clinical setting as a pharmacy technician.
- The most important life-threatening and common drug interactions and contraindications to the use of specific medications. This segment will make mention of drug-disease, drug-drug, drug-dietary supplement, drug-laboratory, and drug-nutrient interactions.
- What do the terms "strength," "dose," and "dosage form" mean, as well as how to determine which route of administration is best for a specific patient and their condition.
- Common and severe side effects of medications, adverse effects, and allergies to specific compounds and active ingredients.
- What some of the indications are to initiate medication and/or a dietary supplement.
- What is meant by "drug stability" in terms of oral suspensions, reconstitutables, vaccinations, injectables, and cold chain processes for insulin.
- What it means to have a medication that has a "narrow therapeutic index."
- A few physical and chemical incompatibilities present when performing non-sterile compounding and reconstitution of medicines.
- The storage of medication, which refers to the temperature ranges, light sensitivity, as well as specific access requirements for specific schedules of medications.

The Federal Requirements Domain

As a pharmacy technician, you need to understand the legalities behind issuing, compounding, and disposing of medications. Now legalities aren't always the most exciting segment to study—we acknowledge that. But it forms a basis for preventing untoward legal action on you, as well as ensures that the patient and environment are protected! Under this domain, you will be expected to know and understand the following concepts:

- What the federal requirements are regarding the handling and disposal of your hazardous and non-hazardous compounds. This section will also cover how to dispose of specific pharmaceutical substances and waste products.
- The legal requirements associated with new controlled substance prescriptions, including their refills and transfers to other generics. Here, the process of DEA controlled substances will also be discussed.
- The legalities behind receiving, storing, loss or theft, labeling, dispensing, and returning of medications.
- The legal concepts that surround restricted drug programs such as pseudoephedrine and codeine. Here, you will also touch on Risk Evaluation and Mitigation Strategies (REMS).
- How the recall process works in terms of the Food and Drug Administration (FDA), as well as the collection and reporting process for medications that have already been dispensed but are being recalled.

The Patient Safety and Quality Assurance Domain

We need to look after our patients! This means we need to be cognizant of the types of medication we dispense. Just imagine what could happen if you give a patient a blood thinner instead of an anti-inflammatory. This results in lethal consequences, which you will be held legally accountable for should it occur.

This domain also refers to expired medications and being hygienic when counting out medications for patients using a counting tray. Yes, we have seen patients have allergic reactions to medications that were counted on trays—simply because the tray was not cleaned properly when their prescription was prepared. This was all a result of the uncleaned residue being on their medication. A few more aspects to consider under this domain include:

- Taking into consideration look-alike and sound-alike medications and the effect they cause when not adhered to.
- How to prevent errors whilst at the pharmacy. This refers to prescription

errors, medication errors, practice errors, leading and trailing zeros, error-prone abbreviations, and the use of barcodes.

- Pharmacy-related issues that require a pharmacy technician to intervene. These circumstances include Drug Utilization Review (DUR), recommended Over-the-Counter (OTC) medications to have in stock, and therapeutic substitution of specific medicines. Patient factors such as post-immunization follow-up, specific medication allergies, as well as how to promote patient adherence to medication will also be covered under this domain.

- How to report instances such as dysfunctional product packaging and possible near misses in the quality assurance process, as well as how to conduct and implement a Root Cause Analysis (RCA).

- The different types of errors that can be discovered on a prescription. This includes but is not limited to early refills, incorrect doses or dosage forms, the incorrect patient, as well as the incorrect medication being prescribed.

- The importance of hygiene within the pharmacy workplace, as well as the cleaning standards that need to be upheld. This includes how to wash your hands correctly, the donning and doffing of Personal Protective Equipment (PPE) when necessary, and ensuring frequent cleaning of counting trays, countertops, and any equipment that is being used.

The Order Entry and Processing Domain

As a pharmacy technician, you won't only be dealing with medications that are in containers. You will also be required to mix antibiotics, make emulsions, and prepare a bunch of non-sterile medicines for your patients. However, there is quite a lot of administration that is behind this process. So, to help you feel better equipped, this is what you are expected to be competent in:

- You need to have a clear understanding of what it means to compound a non-sterile product, how to ensure it is safe for use, as well as what a non-sterile product actually is. Here, you will be taught about ointments, liquids, creating a mixture, as well as how to compound suppositories and enemas.

- Have knowledge regarding how to understand "prescription speak." This includes: what BID and TDS mean, the symbols used for days' supply, quantity, and dose, as well as the formulas needed to calculate proportions, concentrations, and dilutions of medications where necessary.

- The different types of equipment needed to ensure maximal delivery of the medication into the patient's body. Here, you will touch on the use of spacers as well as injectable syringes.
- How to identify the lot number of medications. Here, you will be expected to also be able to locate the expiration date of medicines and their National Drug Code (NDC) number.
- Understanding the procedures related to returning medication dispensed by the pharmacy technician, as well as how to perform a credit return. You will also be taught the concept of reverse distribution in this domain.

What Are the PTCB Eligibility Requirements?

Now although it may seem rather simple to just take an exam, it is not like that at all. As for each certification from a well-renowned board, there is more to simply writing an exam. To apply for certification with the PTCB, you need to do the following over and above passing the exam:

- Need to have undergone PTCB-recognized education and completed PTCB coursework or have obtained a sufficient amount of work experience to supplement the completion of the PTCB-accredited training program.
- Disclosure of all criminal acts, both current and previous, to the State Board of Pharmacy.
- Comply with all of the policies that are applicable to obtaining the PTCB certificate.

Before continuing to a few study hacks, let's explain what is meant by either studying a PTCB-approved course or obtaining work experience. Ultimately, for you to successfully fulfill all eligibility requirements, you need to have either completed a PTCB training program or should have worked a minimum of 500 hours of work within the pharmacy practice setting.

How to Ensure Your Studying Habits Are Successful

Many people get the concept of "studying" completely wrong. It is more than just reading a few sentences and making sense of what you are reading. You need to break the bulk of the learning into sizable chunks, which are studied over a few days. Constant cramming, late nights, and energy drinks will most likely result in you not performing as well in the exam as you would've hoped to. Let the following statement sink in: "You are not incapable of doing well; you probably just don't know how to study!"

We are going to give you tips and tricks of the trade, which will ensure that your study methods are up to scratch. This won't only be beneficial for the PTCB exam but also for the rest of your life.

Your first step is discovering which type of student you are. Do you study better by looking at diagrams? How about actually performing the skills instead of just reading about them? These are the types of questions you will answer to understand which type of "studier" you are and how to apply specific study methods that will work for you. So, let's help you identify which one you are:

- Visual: You study better by looking at diagrams, creating colorful notes, and having the ability to link aesthetics with specific content.
- Auditory: You prefer listening to someone explaining it to you. You will also thrive by repeating the work to yourself. An example of what to do here is to summarize your work and explain the summaries to yourself.
- Kinesthetic: You need to have something moving your body at all times in order to assist you in retaining information. Whether it be chewing gum or playing with a "fidget toy," it keeps you focused and attentive.

You also need to remember that although you may be dominant in one specific study style, you could also be dominant in all three. The only way you are going to be able to establish which one is best for you is by trying each one of them out. Now, once you know how best to capitalize on your best-suited study style, it is time to discuss how you can study for the PTCB exam. And yes, you can self-study for the PCTB exam, and we are going to delve into how you can do just that!

Make Sure You Are Using a Good Book to Read From

You want to ensure the reading material you use is easy to understand and explains concepts well. The material you will need to study for the PTCB exam is highly technical and has an immense amount of jargon. After all, this is to be expected; you are entering into a specialist field. You want the resource to use enough jargon so as not to overwhelm you, as this is exactly how the questions are going to be asked in the exam.

In an exam, sometimes the difference between answering the question and deriving the correct answer is actually understanding what is being asked. Thankfully, this study guide is going to assist you in doing that and so much more.

Make Sure to Use the Practice Tests

The practice tests on the PTCB website, as well as those in this study guide, are geared to give test-takers a prospective view of what and how questions will be phrased in the exam. This is also a perfect way to see if you are ready to tackle the actual exam!

With these kinds of exams, it is very rare that questions are reused, but the chances of this happening are not impossible. We also recommend only doing the practice tests after you have studied and completed all of the required content. It is only in this way that you will be able to have a realistic view of how prepared you are for the exam. It will also show you in which areas your knowledge is not sufficient, prompting you to spend a bit more time on certain topics.

Do Copious Amounts of Research about the Exam

Although the exam and its contents have been summarized and included in this guide, some things aren't included that still remain helpful. Yes, this sounds rather counterintuitive, but we are talking about the lived experiences of people who have failed the tests and then passed on a later attempt.

Complete a PTCB Training Program

By completing a training program that is PTCB-recognized, you are allowing yourself to gain experience that is imperative to pass the exam. Yes, people have passed the exam by just self-studying the content; however, PTCB training programs were designed to make you feel more confident in taking the exam. In these programs, you are trained by the same people that set the exam. Basically, you are given some inside information about what the exam will be like.

However, it is important to reiterate that as of 2020, you need to either have completed 500 hours in order for you to write the PTCB exam purely through self-study. If you have no work experience, completing a PTCB-recognized training program through either a local university or an online school for pharmacy technicians is compulsory.

Be as Hands-On as Possible

It is important to get some form of work experience, even if you are doing a PTCB-recognized training course. This is recommended even more if you use a more kinesthetic-dominant learning and studying style.

As you acquire work experience, you will find that your technical knowledge will become solidified. Sometimes the only way to really concretize concepts is through applying them in real-life situations. This will add a completely new dimension to your thought processes, ensuring that you are even more prepared for the exam.

Creating Your Own Personalized Study Regimen

You know yourself better than anyone. So, who can really make a better study schedule for you than you? The core of your schedule should be based on you knowing your limits and capabilities. If you are one who can only study one month before an exam, then use that as the basis to construct your study schedule. However, you can never go wrong by reviewing notes and knowledge based on real-life work experiences where you felt uncertain.

As you go through the previous PTCB exam papers, put the time in your study schedule to create your own extra questions. Make them difficult and force your mental domain to grow! This is the best way for you to be flexible in understanding the content, especially if they decide to throw you a curveball or two in the exam.

Creating Allocated Study Time Slots

You now understand how you study, as well as how long you need to study in advance. But, how do you structure your day? What many do to not get bored, amongst other reasons, is to divide the topics across different study slots on different days. For instance, doing 1-hour study sessions followed by a 15-minute break is an almost bulletproof approach to ensuring study slots are not too long and boring.

For example, doing pharmacology for two time slots on a Monday, followed by another hour on the federal requirements, ensures variability whilst knocking bits of more than one knowledge domain out of the park.

Make Sure to Take a Break

It is scientifically proven that overstudying is hazardous to both your study habits as well as your overall health. Many students make the mistake of minimal sleep, copious amounts of energy drinks, and little to no exercise. Remember, your brain is like a muscle; it needs time to rest before being able to function optimally again.

Use your scheduled study breaks to do some stretches, take a breather, do some mindfulness practices, have a snack, or make a warm/cold beverage. You will most likely feel more relaxed and confident in your ability to understand new material. Better yet, you may even have heightened clarity on topics you thought you already understood completely.

Rinse and Repeat the Cycle

Repeat your own study cycle as much as you feel you need to. But that doesn't mean not leaving room for alterations. As you get closer to the test date, you may find you're substituting time you would've spent exercising with more study time. If this works for you, then go for it! If you find your study periods are too long, or you need longer study breaks to really restore your brain, make the alterations, and test it out.

You need to be comfortable with the study schedule you have created. The more comfortable you are, the more knowledge you will be able to absorb and retain.

Get Ready for Test Day

As your exam day arrives, you will most likely have times when your anxiety gets the better of you. This is okay and completely normal. The key is having a healthy way to deal with your anxiety. Whether it is listening to your favorite music or watching an episode of a series, knowing what works for you will be imperative, especially as your exam date gets closer and closer.

On the day of your exam, make sure you had a good six to eight hours of sleep the night before. Make sure you eat a good breakfast, looking over some final minute concepts before traveling to your testing center. Psych yourself up by listening to music, chatting with your family, or explaining some last-minute concepts to a friend. The better the mood you are in for your exam, the better you will do.

A quick word on renewing your pharmacy technician certification. After you have passed your exam, depending on which state you are in, you will need to undergo a recertification process which will typically include approximately 20 hours of continued education. There is also a fee for this process, and if your certification lapses, a higher fee and more practical hours will be required to reinstate it.

Studying for the PTCB exam is not easy, but it is definitely doable. You now have a key understanding of what the PTCB exam is, what you can expect, as well as the topics you will be tested on. Now for the fun part, going through the content of the PTCB exam!

Chapter Two: Medications

Now we're going to tap into the different knowledge domains, starting with the most heavily weighted one. In this chapter, we are going to study what generic and brand names are, as well as how medications are classified. We will then go into a few pharmacological terms, such as therapeutic equivalence, drug interactions, contraindications, dietary stability, and the difference between side effects and adverse effects. We will then look at some of the indications of which medications and dietary supplements can be prescribed, ending with the storage of medications and potential incompatibilities when needing to reconstitute a non-sterile compound.

Without further ado, let's get you one step closer to becoming a pharmacy technician!

Names and Classifications of Medications

There are two main types of medication names. These are your generic names and your brand names. As a future pharmacy technician, it is imperative that you understand the difference between these two terms. Many healthcare professionals use these two terms interchangeably; however, some doctors may require that no generics are given at all.

Generic Names

A generic medication is one where the same active ingredient of medication is present, but the tablet or capsule is manufactured by a different company. Generic medications are typically much cheaper than those offered by the original (i.e., brand name) manufacturer.

Getting to produce generics is a process on its own. Many manufacturers have patented their brand name, which typically extends over a period of approximately 20 years. After this time period, other pharmaceutical companies are able to manufacture the medication.

When referring to a medication by its generic name, you may find other people refer to it by its chemical name (i.e., its active ingredient). These two terms are interchangeable.

Brand Names

Based on the generic name definition, you probably know that the brand name refers to the originally produced medication. Although manufacturers will usually advertise the brand name when referring to generic drugs, one needs to remember that one generic drug may have many different brand names. This will be based on different formulations of the same active ingredient, as well as which manufacturer it comes from.

You will be able to identify the brand name as its first letter is always capitalized. This is how you know that it is patented by a specific manufacturer! You will need to be familiar with both generic and brand names when studying the top 200 medications. The reason for this is that they are the most common medications you will be working with in practice as a pharmacy technician.

The Classification System of Medication

As with any system, there is a method to the madness behind the multiple medication names that end with the same suffix. The pharmaceuticals you interact with are classified into "drug classes" that are dependent on how they work (i.e., their mechanism of action) and the way they affect the body.

Many generic names may have the same suffix. For example, medications that end with   -olol, such as propranolol and atenolol, are part of a class known as "beta blockers," which act by decreasing a patient's blood pressure. A few more suffix examples include:

- -pril, which refers to your ACE inhibitors.
- -one, which refers to your corticosteroids.
- -am, which refers to your benzodiazepines.
- -statin, which refers to your cholesterol-lowering medications, referred to medically as HMG-CoA reductase inhibitors.

The same concept can be used when we focus on the prefix of different medications. For example, the prefix cef/ceph refers to a drug class known as "cephalosporins," which are antibiotics effective against bacterial infections. Some examples of this drug class include cephalexin, ceftriaxone, and cefpodoxime.

Therapeutic Equivalence

When we refer to two medications as being "therapeutically equivalent," we are saying that they perform the exact same action on the body. Ultimately, they will have the same clinical effect and safety profile. However, your therapeutic equivalence can only be established after following strict criteria as stipulated by the Food and Drug Administration (FDA).

Therapeutic equivalence has many different terms under its umbrella. Examples of these terms include pharmaceutical equivalents, pharmaceutical alternatives, as well as therapeutic equivalents. When we look at the legal side of things, if a generic medication is therapeutically equivalent to the brand name, it must be swapped out.

Common and Life-Threatening Drug Interactions and Contraindications

There are so many different classes of medication that exist. With that in mind, one can expect that when two different classes of drugs are taken together that there is a chance they will interact with either each other or your body. But, because there are so many different things a drug can interact with, the effect that the drug interaction will have on your body will range in severity from being rather mild to life-threatening.

Although we know about most of the drug interactions that can happen, there is always a possibility that a patient may react in a different way when two different drug classes are taken when compared to someone else. This is why it remains so important to always ensure a patient is educated on what the more common effects of a drug interaction can be and when they need to urgently go to a hospital for more intense and vigorous management.

A Drug-Disease Interaction

This form of interaction is when a specific drug is used for one disease, but it ends up worsening or causing an exacerbation in another disease. An example of this is seen with the use of ibuprofen, an anti-inflammatory under the Non-Steroidal Anti-Inflammatory Drug (NSAID) class. Used for pain, if given to a patient who is going through heart failure, its characteristic retention of fluid could end up resulting in a worsening of the heart failure.

However, it is important to mention that this won't necessarily be the case in all patients. Depending on the degree of heart failure that is present as well as which dose of ibuprofen is used, if the patient tolerates the ibuprofen well, it can be continued. However, if the heart failure starts to worsen, then alternative medications should be used.

A Drug-Drug Interaction

These are interactions that occur between two or more prescription drugs. As a pharmacy technician, you will need to think of any possible serious or life-threatening interactions that can occur and call the prescribing practitioner to change the class of the drug. Seeing multiple different prescribing practitioners and taking multiple medications that are dispensed from multiple pharmacies will increase your risk of developing a drug-drug interaction.

An example of this type of interaction is the concomitant use of omeprazole, a Proton Pump Inhibitor (PPI), and clopidogrel, an antiplatelet medication. This interaction due to omeprazole's enzyme inhibition results in increased reactivity of platelets, ameliorating the intended effect of clopidogrel. The result of this interaction can be the development of a myocardial infarction (i.e., a heart attack).

A Drug-Dietary Supplement Interaction

One of the most common interactions within this category is with drugs and St. John's Wort, which is used to combat many different mental conditions. However, in patients who are on warfarin, a blood thinner, it has actually not only increased the risk of life-threatening bleeding but has also resulted in heightened levels of depression and anxiety. Another example is individuals who use copious amounts of Vitamin E, which, when combined with warfarin, will also result in life-threatening bleeds.

A Drug-Nutrient Interaction

This category of interactions is based on the vitamins, minerals, and nutrients you would obtain from food. This differs from the "dietary supplement" category of interactions in that it is not supplements but rather just one's everyday food intake. It is important that you understand this difference before moving forward.

One of the main instigators in this category of interactions is calcium, typically found in milk products. When it interacts with the fluoroquinolone class of antibiotics (i.e., with active ingredients such as ciprofloxacin), it will decrease the absorption of the antibiotic and will, in some cases, render it completely ineffective. Usually, this will necessitate an increase in the dose of the antibiotic that is administered, especially if ingesting dairy products containing calcium is unavoidable.

What Is a Contraindication?

A contraindication is when a medication is to be completely avoided, as should it be used, the patient's life may be in danger. A very basic example of a contraindication would be any patient taking aspirin—should they have a bleeding disorder. Why is this? Well, aspirin acts on our platelets, preventing clotting and promoting bleeding. You can just imagine the life-threatening implications excessive bleeding can have on someone with a bleeding disorder.

Another common contraindication would be giving a patient a penicillin class of antibiotics when they are known to be allergic to it. This can result in anaphylaxis, a severe immune response with a high mortality rate if the patient is not in a medical facility for immediate treatment and assistance.

Medication Specifications and Calculations

In this subsection, we are going to look at how medications are prepared, the different ways they can be administered, as well as what is meant by the duration of a drug's therapy. We will also be tackling the different types of calculations you will most likely face as a pharmacy technician. Now that you understand what can happen with the different drugs within the body, we are going to shift our focus to how we ensure the chosen drug actually gets into the body to perform its intended action.

The Strength/Dose of a Drug

The strength of a drug can be referred to as the amount of active drug that is present within any particular dosage form. You can usually find what the strength is by looking for an amount that is expressed as either milligrams (mg) or micrograms (mcg). In rare cases, you may even find that nanograms (ng) are used. It is important to always know how to convert mg to mcg, mcg to ng, and vice versa. For example, if you have a prescription that refers to 0.025 mg of levothyroxine, you need to know that it is the same as 25 mcg. The manufacturer's packaging may refer to the 25 mcg and not necessarily the 0.025 mg.

Now although the strength present in a capsule or tablet for oral use is represented as above, for a liquid, the strength will most likely be represented as the amount of milligrams or micrograms in a specific amount of liquid. For example, a specific medication may say there is 125 mg of paracetamol in 5 ml of the liquid. These are typically represented in teaspoons and tablespoons, as these are most commonly used to administer liquids.

Now if we are thinking of the amount of active ingredient that is present within a cream, gel, or ointment, the amount present will most likely be represented in grams (g).

The Dosage Form of a Drug

The dosage form of a drug can be referred to as its physical form. For example, a drug can be present in a tablet, capsule, patch, cream, nasal spray, or even an inhaled aerosol. However, a dosage form that always requires patient counseling is that of an emulsion. The main reason education is required is that an emulsion has two varying densities sitting on top of one another. Thus, it needs to be shaken in order for particles to be dispersed throughout the entirety of the dosage form. This will ensure the correct measurement will have the correct amount of active ingredient present.

There are also many different dosage forms present for the same drug. An example of this is paracetamol which exists as a tablet, a capsule, in a syrup form, as well as an intravenous infusion.

The Administration Routes of a Drug

A drug's route of administration is how it enters the body. These routes of administration can be divided into two broad categories, namely enteral and parenteral. Enteral refers to all types of medication and dosage forms taken by the mouth. Parenteral refers to the main routes of administration:

- inhalation (i.e., through breathing into your lungs)
- oral (i.e., taken by mouth)
- nasal (i.e., via the nose)
- rectal (i.e., via your rectum)

- vaginal (i.e., via a woman's vagina)
- topical (i.e., applied onto the skin's surface)
- transdermal (i.e., applied via a carrying vessel such as a patch with the aim of crossing the skin)
- intramuscular (i.e., injected into the muscle)
- intravenous (i.e., injected via a vein, bypassing the metabolism of the liver and entering straight into the bloodstream)

As a pharmacy technician, it is your duty to make sure the patient knows exactly how the administration of a dosage form needs to be done. For example, you cannot have a patient swallowing a suppository that is intended for rectal use. Not only do you compromise the patient's safety, but also the drug's absorption and action.

Special Administration Requirements and Handling Instructions of Drugs

Some medications need to be stored in a specific manner or environment until they are to be used. An example of this is insulin used for diabetic patients, which needs to be stored in a refrigerator between zero to four degrees Celsius. This is referred to as cold chain storage.

Some medications are also placed in amber glass bottles to prevent condensation of droplets should the bottle be placed in the sun. Should the medication have been placed in the wrong type of packaging, the handling and effectiveness of the drug would be compromised.

In terms of handling specific dosage forms, care needs to be ensured. An example of this is suppositories. It is imperative that gloves are worn as the physical form of the suppository. They can be compromised should we touch them using our own hands. Not only is our body temperature high enough to melt the suppository, but by touching it without gloves and inserting it into the rectum, you are introducing bacteria and other infective microorganisms into the body.

The Duration of a Drug's Use

The duration of a drug's use, also referred to as the "duration of drug therapy," is the total length that the drug will be used. This will be dependent on the patient's diagnosis, as well as whether the condition is acute or chronic in nature. For instance, if a patient is a type one diabetic, they will need to take insulin multiple times per day for the rest of the patient's life. This can be contrasted with the use of an antibiotic for an acute bacterial infection where the duration of treatment, although multiple times per day, will most likely extend between five days and two weeks.

Now it is important that you always educate patients on why they need to adhere to the duration of their therapy. If we look at a chronic condition such as type one diabetes, should the patient not take their insulin and eat a bunch of sweet things, they could become hyperglycemic (i.e., have too much sugar in their bloodstream) and enter into a diabetic coma. In the case of antibiotics, if the duration of therapy is not upheld, your body can actually develop resistance to specific antibiotics. This is a growing problem in today's day and age, and one always needs to follow the guidelines of antibiotic stewardship.

Calculations Performed as a Pharmacy Technician

As a pharmacy technician, you will find yourself making calculations using your basic arithmetic, as well as complex formulas. But, in this case, practice makes perfect! The more comfortable you become with performing calculations, the more likely it will start to become second nature, and you won't even need a calculator to double-check your conversions. Here are a few of the basic calculations we recommend you have memorized:

- One milliliter (ml) is the same as 20 drops
- One teaspoon (tsp) is the same as 5 ml
- One tablespoon (tbsp) is the same as 15 ml
- One kilogram (kg) is the same as 2.2 pounds (lbs)
- One inch (in) is the same as 2.54 centimeters (cm)
- One ounce (oz) is the same as approximately 30 ml
- One pint (pt) is the same as 473 ml

After you have these conversions memorized, we'd recommend you go over the conversions of the metric system as we've discussed before. Here we are referring to examples such as one liter (L) which is the same as 1000 ml, as well as one mg, which is the same as 1,000 mcg. Having a basic understanding of decimals, number rounding, proportions, percentages, ratios, and Roman numerals is worthwhile and will only add to your competence as a future pharmacy technician.

Side Effects, Adverse Effects, and Allergies

When anyone takes medication, they are at risk of developing an unwanted effect. However, it will happen with some patients and not with others. Some may experience nausea and vomiting, others will experience dizziness and blurred vision, and many will not experience anything at all. It is all about your personal factors, such as your genetics, weight, age, and gender, and how they interact with the medication that you take. One needs to also remember that for some patients, that which is considered negative may be positive for them. An example of this is weight loss and hair growth, which some patients may actually benefit from.

The Side Effects of Drugs

Typically, one is able to predict the different side effects that may occur by having an in-depth understanding of how the drug works. But you do get effects that do not correlate with the intended action of a drug, which is considered unwanted. When we look at some of the common side effects that may present when a patient takes particular drugs, they include:

- headaches
- nausea
- vomiting
- diarrhea
- dizziness

Now although many of these side effects will most likely go away, some will persist as long as the drug in question is being used. It is also noteworthy to remember that the side effects portrayed by a specific drug will most likely differ based on the dose used, the dosage form it exists in, as well as the chosen route of administration.

The Adverse Effects of Drugs

An adverse effect of a drug can be seen as a more severe side effect and will most likely result in you needing to discontinue the use of a specific medication. The effect could even become so severe that you may need to go to the hospital to receive emergency medical attention.

Another way to look at an adverse effect is that it is one which will negatively impact a person's quality of life, overall well-being, and disease management. For example, although with the use of simvastatin, a cholesterol-lowering drug, common side effects such as muscle pain and cramping can be present, a severe adverse effect known as rhabdomyolysis can occur. This effect is where simvastatin causes the breakdown of muscles, decreasing your muscle bulk as well as producing dark urine.

Allergies to Drugs

When a patient shows an allergy to a drug, it is often one which cannot be predicted. The reason for this is that the type of response our immune systems cause will be different when comparing people together. With an allergic reaction accounting for 10% of all side effects a drug can have, we need to remember that an allergic reaction can be life-threatening.

Typically, we would refer to a severe allergic reaction as anaphylaxis, where a patient who has most likely taken an antibiotic will present with hives, swelling of both the face and/or throat, wheezing due to the inability to breathe optimally, and worse case scenarios, death. However, it is not only the active ingredient a patient can have an anaphylactic reaction toward. When we look at what makes up a dosage form, it is the active ingredient, as well as the "excipients." Now the excipients are what make up the bulk of the tablet and assist the tablet in looking like an actual tablet.

Some tablets or preparations may use specific dyes or contain gluten, which could result in anaphylaxis for a specific patient. It is also always important to ask a patient whether they have ever had an allergy before, what happened due to the allergy, and what caused the allergy. For some, an allergic reaction may just be an itchy rash that can be treated with a topical or oral antihistamine.

Indications of Medications and Dietary Supplements

When we take a look at the indication for the initiation of medication or dietary supplements, it is the reason why the patient needs to be given said medication or supplements. But, these indications need to be in keeping with the standards set by the FDA, which include all of the different indications that medications and dietary supplements can be prescribed or recommended for.

However, a specific drug's dosage and duration of use may be different based on the indication for which it has been prescribed. An example of this is sertraline, with the brand name Zoloft®, which is an antidepressant that can be prescribed at a dose of 25 mg once a day for patients suffering from Posttraumatic Stress Disorder (PTSD), and then at a dose of 50 mg once a day for patients diagnosed with Major Depressive Disorder (MDD).

In terms of dietary supplements and their indications, it is always advised that they only be initiated on the basis of low blood levels of certain vitamins.

One last term that needs to be discussed under this section is the term "off-label use." What this term refers to is the use of a medication outside of the indications present in the FDA's legend, but it is still a success in treating a particular patient's concern. For example, patients with difficulty falling asleep may find that amitriptyline, an anti-depressant, help them fall asleep quicker despite them not being diagnosed with any mental condition.

Drug Stability

As a pharmacy technician, you need to always ensure that the medication you are issuing to a patient has had its integrity maintained and that it is safe for the patient to use. Within the pharmacy realm, there is a misconception that specific medications and formulations cannot spoil. This is not true. Medications can spoil, and it is our duty as healthcare professionals to ensure that the storage and handling of the medications are of such a nature that, when used, only the expected effect occurs.

When a medication becomes spoiled or has its expiry date exceeded, the drug becomes unstable, leading to its potency becoming compromised. This means that you can unintentionally underdose or overdose your patient. This is quite a gamble on the patient's health, but to prevent this from happening, we are going to jump into a few rules that should be followed when handling and storing specific dosage forms and types of medication.

The Stability of Oral Suspensions

An oral suspension is usually supplied by the pharmaceutical manufacturer as a bottle with a powder inside. This promotes the stability of the medication before it is reconstituted using sterile water. Typically, the powders are stable at room temperature. However, as soon as they are mixed with sterile water, they need to be given a "use by" date. An example of this is when the reconstitution of an amoxicillin powder occurs, it needs to be used within 14 days and is recommended to be stored in the refrigerator.

Another helpful hint regarding oral suspension is always shaking it well before use, even if it has been in the fridge. Sometimes, the powder may create sediment at the bottom of the bottle, which you want to reconstitute before administering the next dose of the medication. This will ensure you are getting the correct amount of active ingredient per unit measurement that has been prescribed.

One also needs to remember that the stability of an oral suspension also depends on how much sterile water the powder is reconstituted with. Use too much, and the concentration of the active ingredient may be too little to cause its desired effect. The contrast is also true!

The Stability of Insulin

It does not matter which insulin a patient is using. Before it is used, all insulins need to be stored in the refrigerator. The cold chain is what will keep the insulin stable until it is used. However, when unused insulin cartridges/pens remain in the fridge, their expiry dates need to always be checked. The last thing you want to do is give a patient expired insulin to use!

Now, let's chat about what happens when the insulin is outside of the fridge and being used by the patient. Depending on the type of insulin the patient is using, the stability of the insulin will remain for a set time period. For example, the insulin aspart (NovoLog) has stability at room temperature for up to 28 days. This is in comparison to the insulin detemir (Levemir), which is stable for longer at room temperature, coming in at 42 days.

It is always important at every visit to make sure that patients are comfortable with injecting themselves with insulin. Some patients may not be doing it correctly, resulting in an uncontrolled glucose level that can cause the patient severe harm.

The Stability of Reconstitutables

The difference between an oral suspension and a reconstitutable is that the latter is supplied as just a dry powder. It is not present in a bottle given by the manufacturer. But, it follows the same process of being a dry powder and needing to be reconstituted with the addition of a diluent. Here, it is noteworthy to mention that although sterile water is usually used, normal saline (i.e., 0.9% NaCl) can also be used in some specific cases.

An example of an antibiotic that comes in a dry powder form is vancomycin, requiring its vial to be reconstituted with a diluent prior to it being added to the intravenous (IV) infusion bag. Some topical reconstitutables may need to be adequately mixed with an aqueous cream base in order for them to have the desired effect.

The Stability of Injectables

Although you get some injectables that are commercially available and can be dispensed to a patient who has a valid prescription, there are, however, some that can only be administered when the patient is either in a hospital or in a doctor's office. As a pharmacy technician, it is your duty to ensure that the stability of the injectables is of maximal standard and that the expiration date has not passed. How the stability and expiration date of the injectables were determined was based on the manufacturer's safety and testing data that was obtained during the drug's testing phase.

With many injectables needing reconstitution and others stable in amber glass vials, as a pharmacy technician, you will always need to remain abreast with the data that indicates when a drug's stability is compromised. An example of an injectable is ceftriaxone, which, when reconstituted, is only stable at room temperature for 24 hours. Thus, it needs to be administered intramuscularly at this time.

The Stability of Vaccines

Vaccines are somewhat fragile and can become unstable rather quickly. When we look at the inadequate storage and handling practices of vaccines, if not adhered to, it can result in a loss of money and inventory, as well as a poor protection profile of patients who require the vaccine.

Now with there being different types of vaccines, it is important to know that your live and attenuated vaccines need to be stored in a refrigerator where the temperature is between 35 and 46 degrees Fahrenheit. However, some vaccines, such as Zostavax, need to be stored in the freezer right up until it is to be administered.

To ensure that the stability of all vaccines is adhered to, it is important to administer the vaccines as soon as it is removed from either the refrigerator or freezer. This will also ensure that no untoward reactions will occur as a result of the instability of the vaccine.

Medications with a Narrow Therapeutic Index (NTI)

As we delve into the different types of medications, some are safer than others. We usually classify the safety of medication based on their "therapeutic index." This is basically where we look at the effect that small differences in a drug's dose have on the human body. More specifically, these effects are usually serious organ failures and adverse drug effects that can result in disability, incapacity, or are life-threatening in nature.

Some of the more common types of medications that have a narrow therapeutic index include warfarin, theophylline, lithium, and phenytoin. Patients on these medications will require regular blood tests to ensure that the concentration of these drugs in their blood is within normal values. Where above, immediate dose reduction is necessary.

Another way to explain a drug's therapeutic index is by asking, "If I took one too many tablets by accident, should I be worried, and if so, how worried should I be?"

Physical and Chemical Incompatibilities Related to Non-Sterile Compounding and Reconstitution

As a pharmacy technician, you always want to ensure that the quality of the medication you compound or reconstitute is always pristine. However, in some cases, whether it be a person-related error or something wrong with the ingredients, the end result can be an unsuitable product. This could either be a physical or chemical incompatibility. Let's go into a bit more detail about the difference between the two.

Physical Incompatibilities

Typically, a physical incompatibility can be seen with the naked eye. However, sometimes it can be very difficult to detect. To ensure that an incompatibility does not exist, we highly recommend always checking the physical consistency of the end product, making sure it is stable and safe to use. A few signs that there is a possible physical incompatibility include the following:

- You see a precipitate being formed. This is primarily the formation of solid particles that sink to the bottom of a liquid formulation.
- You notice a color change that is different than other times the same compound was created.
- Separation of the ingredients no matter how vigorously you mix.
- An unexpected degree of cloudiness in a liquid you have not noticed before.

However, one great thing about physical incompatibilities is that they can often be corrected. This is either through changing the order of mixing in the ingredients, changing the solvents used, adding or removing a suspending agent, or changing the form of the ingredient that is incorporated. We also recommend going over the concepts of an immiscible, hydrophobic, and hydrophilic mixture. For completeness' sake, also make sure you understand what an emulsifier is and how it is used in compounding.

In some cases, you can change everything, but the medications just won't combine. This is a reality, as some chemical compounds just won't mix together! For example, a well-known example of physical incompatibility is that of calcium and ceftriaxone. When these two are combined together, they form a precipitate. This is why healthcare professionals are taught not to administer these two drugs in the same tubing. Not to mention that the precipitate is lethal should it be administered.

Chemical Incompatibilities

A chemical incompatibility is usually not seen with the naked eye. But, if it is an extreme reaction, physical changes will be noticeable. However, typically these incompatibilities will cause an alteration in the chemical compatibility and makeup of the compounds, which could render the end product either toxic, unstable, or completely inactive. To solidify the concept, let's look at a few of the more common chemical incompatibilities:

- A change in the compounds' pH
- Decomposition or degradation of either of the ingredients

- Hydrolysis of the end product
- The inclusion of an oxidation-reduction reaction

Now, these are all biochemical concepts you should already be familiar with when you did chemistry in high school. However, we highly recommend doing a bit of a touch-up on these concepts so that you can really understand the nuances of chemical incompatibilities.

If you get stuck and need a bit more practice in solidifying the concepts of physical and chemical incompatibilities, there are a bunch of quizzes online that will assist you in becoming rather astute in identifying the differences.

The Proper Storage of Medications

The way in which many medications are stored is not only to maintain their physical and chemical compatibility. In many cases, there is a bunch of legislation that governs how different medications, based on either scheduling status or abuse potential, should be stored. We're going to pack all of this into a quaint little package by discussing the two concepts separately.

The Temperature Ranges of Medications

Most medications you will interact with as a pharmacy technician will be stable and of the desired quality at room temperature. Now room temperature is 25 degrees Celsius or between 68 and 77 degrees Fahrenheit. With that being said, some drugs need to remain refrigerated. These are usually kept between 2 and 8 degrees Celsius or between 36 and 46 degrees Fahrenheit. There are even drugs that need to be stored in the freezer at temperatures that are between -10 and -25 degrees Celsius or between -13 and 14 degrees Fahrenheit.

But what happens if there is no specific storage requirement that exists on the medication's packaging? Well, we will then assume that it is to be kept at room temperature.

The Light Sensitivity of Medications

Believe it or not, some medications are very sensitive to light. Scientifically, we refer to them as being "photosensitive." Typically, what will happen should these medications be placed in the sun is that they will degrade. Now, as a pharmacy technician, when you count out pills for a prescription, you have the choice of which storage method to utilize.

Different methods of medication storage can yield different results. This is why it is advised that if the medication comes from the manufacturer in an amber bottle, it should be dispensed in an amber bottle. Now, these bottles are rather special as they deflect light rays, maintaining the stability of the medication. An example of a drug that needs to be in an amber container is nitroglycerin, a drug used to aid in symptomatic management in patients with coronary artery disease (CAD).

The Restricted Access of Medications

Some drugs are considered to be controlled substances and need to be kept within designated areas of access in the pharmacy. These medications may need to be in a locked cupboard that is only accessible by certain staff members. It also goes without mentioning that care needs to be taken to ensure that these controlled substances are not accessible by children, adolescents, and other members of the general public.

Controlled substances are usually categorized, all with their own specific rules and regulations that need to be followed. For those within categories C-III to C-V, which will include lorazepam, zolpidem, and buprenorphine, the storage is different based on the pharmacy's preference. Some pharmacies will keep it locked away; others will keep it on the shelves in the dispensary.

Medications that are within the C-II category are classified as having a high abuse potential and will always need to be kept in a cupboard that is secured with a lock and key. Some pharmacies even find that using a vault or cage is of benefit. Examples of medications in this category include your opioid class of drugs, such as oxycodone and fentanyl. Your drugs that are used to treat ADHD will also be present in this category!

You have now successfully completed the "Medications" segment of the PTCB exam! This is definitely something you can celebrate. At this point, you should feel comfortable in identifying the generic and brand names of medication, as well as understanding terms such as therapeutic equivalence and a narrow therapeutic index. You have also gone through the different types of forms that medications can come in and the potential effects, both wanted and unwanted, they can cause.

Remember, this section is weighted the most out of all the four knowledge domains, so you need to make sure you have an in-depth and solid understanding of the concepts we've discussed in this chapter. But it is time to tackle the second knowledge domain—Federal Requirements!

Chapter Three: Federal Requirements

As a pharmacy technician, you will not only need to think about the medications you are providing your patients with. You will also need to take into account the legalities that exist with the different types of drugs you can issue without a prescription, why this is so, and how you can legally dispose of both expired medications and other pharmaceutical waste.

In this segment, we are also going to be discussing the different schedules of medication and in which cases you can transfer a prescription from one pharmacy to another. There will also be a few interesting notes on calculations you may need to do as a pharmacy technician, including what to do in the case of a manufacturer recalling a specific batch of drugs based on compromised safety or physical/chemical incompatibilities.

Although this knowledge domain is only approximately 12.5% of the entirety of your test, it is imperative information that must be known by every pharmacy technician. Laws and regulations can be rather difficult to understand, all the more so because it is a completely different kind of knowledge than what we are used to. But, it isn't impossible to grasp, and we are going to show you how easy it can actually be.

Handling and Disposal of Pharmaceutical Substances and Waste

As a pharmacy technician, you are not only responsible for protecting others when handling hazardous substances. You also need to protect yourself in the process! When you find yourself needing to work or handle hazardous material, especially those that may require personal protective wear, make sure you abide by all the rules. Each pharmaceutical substance that is hazardous will most likely come with a Safety Data Sheet (SDS), which will provide you with substance-specific information regarding the handling, toxicity, and damage the substance can do to your body if you aren't careful.

Hazardous Materials

Let's first tackle what it means when a substance or material is labeled as being "hazardous." This type of material is one that has the potential to cause harm, of varying degrees, to any person that either comes into contact with it or plays an active role in preparing it. Luckily for us, there is the Occupational Safety and Health Administration (OSHA) which has implemented specific standards that act to protect all employees. Yes, that includes other members of staff, who may need to either transport the finished product or the delivery clerks to the different hospital wards.

The standards that OSHA has imposed include a bunch of different procedures that can be followed, which include the total allotted time a worker can be exposed to the substance per day, their maximum exposure limits, employees with specific health conditions that cannot interact with the hazardous substance, and when PPE needs to be donned.

When disposed of, these substances need to be placed in a container that is leakproof and labeled "hazardous drug waste." This is to ensure that no other employees mistake the contents of the container for something else and use it erroneously.

As a pharmacy technician, you will either witness or make mistakes. So, in the case of accidental exposure to a hazardous substance through it either splashing into your eyes, it touching your skin, or the inhalation of fumes, make sure you know where the "rescue equipment" is. For example, all areas that make use of hazardous substances need to have an eyewash station.

All areas should also have a file with all the SDS documents of all hazardous substances, spill kits to help you clean up the area, as well as an incident reporting form that needs to be given to your supervisor. A few examples of these substances include inorganic arsenic, lead, cadmium, benzene, formaldehyde, ethylene oxide, acrylonitrile, and chromium.

Non-Hazardous Materials

Now even though these materials may not pose any direct harm to an individual, they still need to be disposed of correctly. As a pharmacy technician, you need to always keep it at the back of your mind that all types of materials, if handled incorrectly, have the potential to cause harm. Although when using these materials, PPE is not a necessity, handling these materials with care remains your priority.

As healthcare workers, we don't only care about our patients. We also try our best to take care of the environment. With these materials posing a significant risk to the environment should they not be disposed of correctly, their rules regarding disposal should be followed as strictly as hazardous materials. For example, should we just dump these materials down the drain, they could find their way into our waterways and contaminate the water you and I drink. The disposal of non-hazardous materials can take many different forms. Usually, these materials are either disposed of at mass landfill sites or are incinerated.

Typically, you may even find that some of the materials you use can be recycled and composted. Not only will this decrease the amount of greenhouse gas emissions, but it will also save energy, allow for the creation of greener technology, and reduce the necessity for more landfills and combustors.

Pharmaceutical Substances

These substances are those that are used therapeutically to treat or prevent diseases. They include medications or the different ingredients that are used to make them. For example, when we look at the formation of a tablet, the pharmaceutical substances would refer to both the active ingredient and the excipients chosen for use.

There are two main categories under your "pharmaceutical substances." These are, namely, hazardous pharmaceutical substances and non-hazardous pharmaceutical substances. Examples of hazardous pharmaceutical substances include the following drugs: warfarin, tretinoin, methotrexate, phenytoin, and finasteride. Some examples of non-hazardous pharmaceutical substances include atorvastatin, amoxicillin, diphenhydramine, cyclizine, and ranitidine.

With regard to vaccines, there is an extra precaution that needs to be taken. Now, this is not with the vaccine vial itself but more with the process of injecting a patient. Needle-stick injuries are a common method of transferring HIV and hepatitis, and every pharmacy technician needs to be cognizant of this when preparing to inject anyone. It is also important that all syringes and needles that are used in providing the injection are disposed of in an appropriate sharp container. These are typically readily available either throughout the pharmacy or in the hospital wards.

Federal Requirements for Controlled Substance Prescriptions and DEA Controlled Substance Schedules

Federal requirements are always important to abide by. As a pharmacy technician, you need to continually ask yourself whether what you are doing is legal and abides by both your DEA and state laws. Luckily for all of us, these laws and regulations are usually very similar year after year and only ever have very minor changes.

All about Controlled Substances

Your "controlled substances" are those that have an inherently high risk of either being abused by patients or misused. Medications that fall into this category are not only highly regulated by the Drug Enforcement Administration (DEA) but are further classified into different schedules based on their misuse or abuse potential.

In many pharmacies, there are designated areas where these drugs are stored, with the main reasons being to monitor their stock levels more rigidly, as well as remove access to it by the general public. These areas will either be of the locked cabinet variety or a separate vault.

The Movement of Controlled Substances

Medication is moved to the pharmacy from the designated manufacturer. The medication is then moved from the pharmacy personnel to the patient. Both of these transfers are regulated by the DEA. As the substance moves hands, there needs to be a controlled and mediated tracking system. The reason for this is to ensure that the medication is handled correctly and that the chances of unethical practices are minimized. But, depending on whether the prescription is new or not, as well as the scheduling status of the medication on the prescription, the rules regarding movement may differ.

New Prescriptions

For drugs that fall under "Schedule II," the prescription needs to be sent to the pharmacy from the practitioner electronically. Alternatively, a prescription note from the practitioner in a hard copy format will also be accepted. Faxes are used a lot less nowadays; however, they will still be accepted only if the patient is in a hospice or they are classified as being "long-term care" patients.

Should the patient run out of their supply of medications for a specific reason, it is possible to allow the practitioner to call the pharmacy to request a 72-hour emergency supply of medication or however much is needed to combat the described emergency. In these instances, an electronic or hard copy of the prescription needs to be furnished to the pharmacy as soon as possible. This is as per the DEA regulations.

With the current existence of an opioid crisis, one where patients are misusing opioids to the extent that they are becoming addicted to them, the DEA needed to step in. The result of this is a limit of up to 100 morphine milliequivalents (MME) being prescribed per day. The only way to bypass this rule is for there to be a relevant ICD-10 code. The ICD-10 codes system is one where letters and numbers are allocated to a specific disease, allowing medical aids and pharmacies to correlate the medication with the patient's condition.

With prescriptions that contain Schedule II drugs, no alterations are allowed on the prescription. Even if you were to call the practitioner and discuss changes with them, they would need to furnish a new prescription. Usually, depending on which state you plan on practicing in, there is an expiration date of 90 days from the written date of any prescription that is not explicitly stated to contain repeats. Your Schedule II drugs cannot be repeated and are limited to a 30-day supply per fill.

It is noteworthy to mention that only medications that are between Schedule III and Schedule V can be repeated. These classes of drugs have less abuse potential than your Schedule II drugs, and it is for this reason that they can be repeated for a period of six months without needing to furnish a new and legitimate prescription. Pharmacy personnel can also dispense up to a 90-day supply of Schedule III to Schedule V medication.

As a pharmacy technician, especially one who will be dealing with prescriptions, you need to follow both the federal law, as well as the laws stipulated by the state in which you practice. However, in a case where the two are different from each other, you will need to employ your own judgment, instituting the regulation that is stricter.

Refills

Your Schedule II drugs cannot be refilled. We wrote it again because this is one of the main causes of punitive action against pharmacy technicians. It does not matter whether the patient only wants a particular portion of their prescription or whether their health insurance has a specific quantity limit, the amount remaining is forfeited. This means that should the patient have 15 tablets left over, they will need to get another prescription for those 15 tablets.

However, an exception to this rule is that of hospice patients. These patients are able to divide their 30-day-long script into 60 days from the written date. Any medication that has not been obtained after the 60-day period will then be forfeited.

Thankfully, all the medications in the Schedule III to Schedule V category can be refilled a maximum of five times (excluding the original prescription) or over a period of six months.

Regarding your controlled substances, they cannot be refilled earlier than the mandated date. In many cases, a one to two-day period of grace is given from the actual day the refill is due. However, some health insurance may still reject the claim until the actual day on which you are to refill your medication.

The Transfer of a Prescription

Moving is inevitable. You may even find yourself out of town and having forgotten to refill your prescription. But what do you do then? Well, depending on your prescription's scheduling status, you may either need to obtain a completely new prescription, or you can refill your script should the two respective pharmacies share an online database.

Your Schedule II drugs cannot be transferred and will thus need a new prescription. It does not matter whether these two pharmacies share an online database (for example, from one Walgreens to another Walgreens). By law, it is not allowed. However, your Schedule III to Schedule V drugs can only be transferred once. This is only the case should the two respective pharmacies not share an online database. If a common database is used, then the prescription can be transferred until either expires or until all the refills have been used up.

Regarding your Schedule III to Schedule V transfers, you'll need to know that lawfully you can only transfer a script should the patient only require refills. What this means is that if the patient never came to obtain the prescription drugs for the first time, they are not allowed to have the script transferred.

As a pharmacy technician, when you transfer a prescription from one pharmacy to another, you will need to void the original prescription at your pharmacy. You will then need to add a note to the patient's profile stating where the prescription was transferred to and what date this occurred. Remember, if you think you have noted down too little, you most probably have. Always put as much information as possible about any transfers.

The following information needs to be included when you are transferring a prescription:

- When the original date of the prescription was.
- What the initial dispensing date of the prescription was.
- How many refills are still valid for this prescription.
- What the name of the pharmacist is to whom the prescription is being transferred to.
- The name, DEA number as well as the address of the initial pharmacy. This is your pharmacy, also known as the "transferring pharmacy."

DEA Controlled Substance Schedules

The scheduling system that the DEA has implemented is based on the potential that a specific drug can be misused and abused. The drugs with the highest regulation are Schedule I drugs with the highest potential for abuse but do not exist on the market. The reason for this is that they are seen as drugs that are not effective treatments for diseased states and that provide little to no therapeutic benefit.

Your Schedule II drugs have been discussed rather extensively and are the highest regulated drugs that are on the market. As the Schedule number increases, the potential for abuse and misuse decreases. However, as a pharmacy technician, it is important to remember that just because a specific drug isn't highly regulated, it does not mean that it cannot be abused.

Calculations You Should Be Aware Of

With the controlling of prescriptions, there are limitations on both the quantity supplied as well as the number of days that are supplied to the patient. As a pharmacy technician, it is imperative that you are comfortable in calculating the days of supply a prescription is written for. Now seeing that it is typically the pharmacist that is held responsible for ensuring that each prescription that comes through the pharmacy coincides with all federal legislation and state regulations, a pharmacy technician needs to be able to detect inconsistencies before it reaches the pharmacist.

We have discussed the opioid prescription limit of 100 MME. Now if we have more than one drug that contains an opioid on the prescription, the result is cumulative. What this means is that the MME value of one opioid will be added to the other opioid, and the total is not to exceed 100. You will need to know some of the more common MME conversion factors. Here are a few of them:

- Morphine: An MME conversion factor of 1.
- Oxycodone: An MME conversion factor of 1.5.
- Hydrocodone: An MME conversion factor of 1.
- Codeine: An MME conversion factor of 0.15.

To solidify this concept, let's look at an example. Mr. X comes into the pharmacy with a valid prescription. He is prescribed oxycodone 5 mg tablets that are to be taken orally every eight hours. He has been prescribed 84 tablets in total. These are the conversions you will use:

- A total of 84 tablets divided by the frequency (three times per day) = a 28-day supply.
- Each tablet consists of 5 mg of oxycodone and is taken three times per day = a total daily dose of 15 mg of oxycodone.
- Taking the daily dose of oxycodone and multiplying it by oxycodone's MME factor (i.e., 1.5) = a total of 22.5 MME per day.

This prescription is safe to dispense as not only is the opioid content less than 100 MME per day, but the daily limit is also less than the 30-day maximum.

Federal Regulations for Controlled Substances

Controlled substances do not follow your typical "movement" pattern as stipulated above. For instance, it does not matter where the controlled substances are present, there are ethical practices that need to be followed. These standards are put in place to govern the pharmacies, practitioners, as well as manufacturers of the specific drug.

Regulations Associated with Controlled Substances

With the above in mind, two main regulatory bodies govern the regulations pertaining to controlled substances. These are the Drug Enforcement Agency (DEA) and the Food and Drug Administration (FDA).

The DEA

This regulatory agency aims to eliminate illegal practices and the potential for drug diversion within the United States. In accordance with the Comprehensive Drug Abuse Prevention and Control Act of 1970, all of those that are in contact with a controlled substance need to have the ability to provide records that are continuously updated. Regular inventory needs to be taken in order to ensure that no illegal activities and drug diversion are occurring.

The role of every pharmacy technician is to ensure that the pharmacy remains aligned with all federal requirements. With all of these regulations in place, there are specific differences regarding the record-keeping of the different schedules of medications. These are divided into record-keeping practices for Schedule II drugs, those between Schedules III and V, and those that are classified as being non-controlled substances.

It is important to mention that the activities mentioned in this subsection are also commonly known as the Controlled Substances Act of 1970, with both versions being used interchangeably.

All pharmacies and practitioners need to ensure that before they can either prescribe or dispense any type of controlled substance, they need to first register with the DEA. Both the pharmacy and the practitioner will be issued with their own unique DEA number that needs to always remain active for controlled substances to be prescribed and dispensed. Usually, a DEA number can be identified by it containing two letters and seven numbers. The first letter of the DEA number will identify which type of DEA registry document was completed, with the second letter being the first letter of a prescriber's surname.

There is a rather complex way you can go about manually verifying whether a DEA number is actually a true DEA number or not. The manner of doing this is as follows:

- Take the first, third, and fifth numbers and add them together.
- Then take the second, fourth, and sixth numbers and add them together.
- Take the answer you received by adding the second, fourth, and sixth numbers, and multiply it by two.
- Take your answer of the cumulated first, third, and fifth numbers, as well as the answer you just multiplied, and add them together.
- The second digit of your answer should coincide with the prescriber's last digit present in their DEA number.

Over and above ensuring that all federal and state regulations are adhered to, practitioners, pharmacists, as well as pharmacy technicians need to periodically check a patient against the Prescription Monitoring Program (PMP). Not only will you be able to see a patient's complete controlled substance history, but you can also identify whether the patient does doctor shopping (going to many practitioners for multiple prescriptions), has polypharmacy (taking a large amount of different medications), or is constantly obtaining early refills.

The FDA

Now where the DEA focuses on the misuse potential of drugs, the FDA takes it a step further and ensures that all medical devices, biologics, and drugs are safe, efficacious, and of the highest quality. How the drugs are regulated is that each drug needs to go through an FDA approval process before being able to enter the market.

The FDA is also responsible for a few other domains, such as the manufacturing, dispensing, labeling, and postmarket surveillance of all medications, devices (where applicable), and biologicals. There are even some drugs that have a black box warning on them. This is an FDA requirement that has the aim of informing both healthcare practitioners and patients of the possibility of severe adverse effects or life-threatening risks being attributed to the particular drug.

An example of a black box warning is with opioids, whereby the warning alerts everyone to the high risk of addiction, abuse, misuse, as well as respiratory depression, a life-threatening physiological response to a large amount of opioids. This is why the FDA needed to implement the Opioid Analgesic Risk Evaluation and Mitigation (REMS) program.

The REMS program is important as it allows patients to be monitored in time windows where the chance of them developing severe adverse effects is the greatest. This has the added advantage of also ensuring no patient is misusing or becoming dependent on opioids.

With regards to the postmarketing surveillance that the FDA employs, they are present to monitor the concerns regarding the safety and efficacy of those drugs that have recently entered the market. An example of how postmarketing surveillance has impacted the labeling of specific drugs was in 2019 when the FDA required that all opioids needed to have dose tapering instructions on their labels. This was to ensure no adverse events would occur after the abrupt continuation of long-term opioid use. The main reporting program that the FDA uses is MedWatch.

An Overview of the Regulation Categories

As we already know by now, the lifecycle of any controlled substance is filled with many different rules and checkpoints. With each step needing to explicitly comply with all federal and state rules, there is little to no room for error. In addition, if these protocols are not adhered to, and there are no records of how the controlled substances have been handled, you are in big trouble!

Let's take a deeper look at the lifecycle of controlled substances, as well as a few of the schedule-specific rules that exist.

Receiving of Controlled Substances

When we look at Schedule II drugs, upon receiving the order, the responsibility is on the pharmacist to not only verify each item that is being received but also the date the order was received. Usually, this information can be documented on the third copy of the original order form. This third copy is then legally required to be filed and kept within the pharmacy's presence for a period of at least two years.

Regarding Schedule III to V drugs, there are no special requirements. The rules regarding the receiving of non-controlled drugs will apply in these cases.

Storing of Controlled Substances

It is because controlled substances are highly regulated that they need to be stored properly. We've already discussed that your Schedule II drugs need to always be kept under lock and key and cannot share their vault or cabinet with medication of another Schedule. Not only must there be a proper locking mechanism in place, but having multiple cameras positioned around the vault or cabinet is nonnegotiable.

Regarding your Schedule III to V drugs, you can either have them present in their own vaults or have them dispersed amongst the other non-controlled inventory that is in the pharmacy. However, you need to make sure that cameras are also positioned for these drugs to be monitored. The decision on whether to place the Schedule III to V drugs in their own cabinet or on the general shelves is at the discretion of the pharmacist in charge.

Ordering of Controlled Substances

With your Schedule III to V drugs not having any specific ordering requirements, this section will be focusing on the process that Schedule II drugs need to follow.

Your Schedule II drugs need to be ordered through the use of a specific form.

This form is the DEA 222. Handwritten or typed out, this form needs to be completed in a triplicate fashion. The need for this is to enable tracking at various stages of the supply chain. The supplier of the Schedule II drugs is given the top copy, followed by the DEA receiving the middle copy, and the bottom copy is kept by the purchaser. A completed DEA 222 form is only valid for a maximum of 60 days, with only a total of 10 different medications per form allowable. These forms need to be signed by a DEA-registered pharmacist.

Now if you don't have access to a DEA 222, you can use the Controlled Substance Ordering System (CSOS). With a pharmacy needing to apply for eligibility, extra factors such as digital firewalls and extra layers of digital security need to be present. The CSOS system is currently being rapidly adopted as it takes away the need for a paper-based system. It also adds to the convenience aspect associated with running a pharmacy and keeping all the documents neat and accessible when needed.

In October 2019,6 the DEA decided that instead of using a triplicate system, only a single DEA 222 form would be used. As it was being implemented across the US, a period of two years was when both triplicate and single DEA 222 forms were present. However, regarding the single DEA 222 form, the purchaser of the controlled substances needs to keep a copy of the order form and then send the original form to the supplier. In some cases where the pharmacy or the healthcare practitioner is the supplier, a copy of the order form needs to be sent via email to the DEA.

Labeling of Controlled Substances

There are quite a few mandatory inclusions that need to be on a medication's label. However, specifically to the labels of controlled substances, for a label to be compliant with the required federal regulations, the following needs to be present:

- The date that the prescription was filled.
- The name and address of the pharmacy.
- The prescription number.
- The name of the patient.
- The practitioner who prescribed the patient's medication.

- The name of the drug, its strength, as well as its dosage form.
- The quantity that needs to be dispensed, as well as the number of fills the prescription is valid for. The latter is only applicable to drugs that are within the Schedule III to V class.
- Directions for the correct use of the drugs.
- Any extra cautions that need to be taken into consideration.

Over and above these inclusions, the FDA requires that the label always contains a specific warning. This warning should read, "Caution: Federal law prohibits the transfer of this drug to any person other than the patient for whom it was prescribed." This warning was put in practice to ensure patients do not share their medication, especially anti-anxiety and sleeping tablets, with other members of their family.

Dispensing of Controlled Substances

Irrespective of whether the medication is a controlled substance or not, a prescription is only able to be dispensed if it is considered to be valid. It is considered valid if a legitimate medical practitioner has written it for a medical purpose that is within the scope of the practitioner. As a pharmacy technician, you will need to be able to validate prescriptions, as well as ascertain the degree of therapeutic benefit the prescription will supply the patient with. Once all the boxes have been ticked, the medication can safely and legally be dispensed to the patient.

Keeping the above in mind, there are also a few extra boxes that need to be considered. These are as follows:

- A prescription needs to be dispensed to either the patient or any member who is a part of their household. If given to any other person, there is a term change. The medication is then not dispensed but rather distributed to another person.
- As is the case in many pharmacies, a patient would usually have to have some sort of federally-approved identification when picking up their medication. This ensures that the person picking up the medication is indeed who they say they are and limits the chances of drug diversion from occurring.
- For those patients who suffer from pain, some states have imposed

measures to combat the ever-rising opioid epidemic. To do this, they have initiated a maximum of a seven-day supply of opioids to treat acute pain and 30 days to treat chronic pain.

Reverse Distribution of Controlled Substances

The concept of "reverse distribution" refers to instances where a pharmacy will send a specific drug manufacturer all of their outdated drugs, as well as those drug products which are unusable. Usually, this is for the main aim of having the medication processed or safely disposed of.

Controlled substances that are either damaged, outdated, or no longer wanted by either the patient or pharmacy may be destroyed. However, this can only occur after being authorized by the DEA. In order for the approval process to be initiated, a licensed distributor or pharmacy needs to fill in a DEA 41 form. The contents of the form include the following:

- The date and location where the destruction of the controlled substances will take place.
- The chosen method of destruction.
- The name, strength, and dosage form of the controlled substance that is to be destroyed.
- The NDC and quantity that is to be destroyed.
- The details of two employees who will sign off as witnesses to the destruction.

Take Back Programs for Controlled Substances

These programs are fantastic ways to ensure that unwanted and expired medication is safely disposed of. These programs do not have different rules and regulations for whether the medication is a controllable substance or not.

Occurring a few times a year, they are typically hosted at universities or police stations. The substances that are received at these locations are provided voluntarily so that they can be disposed of in the correct manner. The effect of these programs is a safer community, which ensures excess drugs do not end up in erroneous places such as waterways and in the hands of the general public.

Loss and Theft of Controlled Substances

Life happens, and in some cases, a pharmacy may be targeted because it is known to have controlled substances on its premises. In the event that substances that are Schedule II to Schedule V are either lost or stolen, both the DEA as well as the local law enforcement authorities need to be immediately notified.

A DEA 106 form is then filled out by the pharmacist, including all the details of the medication that was stolen from the premises. The DEA is then sent the original form, with the pharmacy retaining a copy of the form for recording purposes. Instances where a small amount of a controlled substance is compromised, such as the spilling of a small amount of liquid or a few tablets breaking, do not constitute a report to the DEA. Only losses that are significant in nature need to have a DEA 106 form filled out.

Federal Requirements for Restricted Drug Programs, Related Medication Processing, and FDA Recall Requirements

There are many instances where patients have been given incorrect medication. Depending on the type of medication given, it can either result in no harm at all or a life-threatening event. There are even some scenarios where a patient who is pregnant or has a particular disease is given a drug that would be contraindicated in this specific patient. It is for this reason that some drugs with the potential to be harmful have strict criteria that need to be fulfilled before the filling of the prescription can be done.

Restricted Drug Programs

Quantity limits, patient tracking, and strict recordkeeping practices are put in place for patients who are using specific medications. Not only can an overdose of specific medications yield catastrophic results, but it also does not reflect too well on the pharmacy, or pharmacy technician, who may have been involved in dispensing the medication to the patient.

Pseudoephedrine

One of the most common drugs that are placed on a restricted drug program is pseudoephedrine. In accordance with the Combat Methamphetamine Epidemic Act of 2005 (CMEA), restrictions have been placed on the sale, storage, and extent of record keeping that is required. However, these extra tasks are not just for pseudoephedrine but also include all medical products that contain either ephedrine or phenylpropanolamine.

One of the requirements under this Act is that a maximum amount of 3.6 grams of this product can be bought per day. This amount then increases to 9 grams over a period of 30 days. It is important to note that this specific weight is based on the amount of base chemical within the formulation and not the overall tablet's strength.

Pseudoephedrine, ephedrine, and phenylpropanolamine need to be stored behind the pharmacy counter, with all patients' details and logbooks being accurately filled in.

Risk Evaluation and Mitigation Strategies (REMS)

These strategies are programs that are run between drug manufacturers and the FDA. These programs aim to limit the amount of inappropriate dispensing that occurs, as well as to protect the patient from the pharmacist/pharmacy technician. Yes, we know that sounds a bit harsh, but sometimes we can be dangerous!

Regarding the contents of the REMS programs, each specific drug will have its own set of criteria that need to be achieved. The criteria can range anywhere from patient education to specific laboratory tests that need to be conducted before a specific drug is initiated. A few extra instructions regarding the safe use of a drug are included in the communication plan between the patient and the healthcare provider.

An example of a drug that is present in a REMS program is isotretinoin. This drug is a part of the retinoid class of drugs and is used to combat severe acne. However, it is teratogenic when given to pregnant women.

Thus, the Isotretinoin Safety and Risk Management Act has instituted measures that ensure that disastrous effects on the fetus do not occur. Legally, a patient will need to have blood tests done as well as undergo rigorous counseling before they can have a prescription given to them. The prescription then needs to be filled within a 7-day window, with a maximum of 30 days after being given to the patient.

Calculations You Are Required to Know

We spoke about pseudoephedrine and the total amount of grams that can be purchased per day and over a 30-day period. We're going to delve into a clinical scenario to assist you in understanding the concept a bit better.

Patient Z is feeling a bit flush and decides to come and get some pseudoephedrine. You have the Pseudoephedrine HCl 30 mg tablets in stock. Each tablet has 24.6 milligrams of base chemical. With each box containing a total of 24 tablets, we will now calculate the total amount of boxes they can legally buy from the pharmacy. This will be done as follows:

- As per the CMEA guidelines, pseudoephedrine has a 3–6 gram limit. This equates to a total of 3,600 milligrams.
- Dividing the 3,600 as the maximum limit by the amount of base chemical in each tablet will give you the maximum amount of tablets you can dispense. Thus, 3,600 milligrams divided by 24.6 milligrams of base chemical per tablet = 146 tablets.
- With each box consisting of 24 tablets, 146 tablets divided by 24 = 6.08. This means that this patient will not be legally allowed to purchase more than six boxes of pseudoephedrine from your pharmacy today.

Recalls of Medication

Sometimes errors in particular drugs are only detected after the drug has already been dispensed to a patient. In these cases, when a manufacturer recalls a specific drug's batch, all patients to whom the drug was dispensed to need to be called and have their drugs removed from their possession. This is why accurate records always need to be kept. At the end of the day, the more accurate your records, the safer your patients will be.

Recall Targets

It does not matter how short or long a drug has been on the market. The FDA reserves the right to recall any medical product at any given time. Should there be any concern regarding the safety of the product, a pharmaceutical manufacturer has the option to voluntarily recall the product.

The Recall Targets of Medications

There are a bunch of reasons why medication can be recalled. Usually, medications are recalled when there is a safety concern. Some examples of reasons for a recall to take place include the identification of impurities in the product, mislabeling of the product, unexpected and unexplained adverse effects, as well as contamination of the product.

The Recall Targets of Medical Devices

When medical devices pose either a health hazard to a patient or are defective, they would usually be recalled. Some of the more common medical devices that have been recalled include insulin pumps, cardiac pacemakers, infusion pumps, and glucose meters. This is not an extensive list, and many more medical devices have been recalled.

The Recall Targets of Medical Supplies

Medical supply manufacturers have, at times, notified the FDA of either faulty components or batches of supplies that are unable to perform their intended use. Examples of these medical supplies include surgical gloves, needles and syringes, catheters, and sterile water solutions. Usually, an example of such a recall would be based on either a syringe that has had its measurement markings erroneously printed or your surgical gloves that have a powdered residue present.

The Recall Targets of Supplements

Supplements have the potential to pose health risks for the same reasons you would find with your prescription and OTC medication recalls. Some of the more common reasons for a supplement to be recalled include either an increased or decreased potency, incorrect labeling of the product, the presence of ingredients that have not been declared, and possible contamination.

Categories of Recalls

There are different categories of recalls that exist. When a recall is issued, the FDA will place the recall in a Class to indicate the importance of the recall. There are three different recalls that the FDA can impose. They are as follows:

- Your Class I recalls are the most severe. Here the medication that is being recalled will have the potential to cause life-threatening adverse effects and, in worst-case scenarios, death. A common cause of a Class I recall is when one drug is found to have been mislabeled as another drug.
- A Class II recall will occur when the drug has the potential to cause a reversible and temporary adverse effect. Usually, a Class II recall will also include your drugs having a small chance of causing a serious adverse event.
- Your least severe type of recall is your Class III recalls. The drugs recalled within this Class will most likely not cause any adverse effects, but they need to be recalled because of the compromised therapeutic efficacy.

This chapter has been very detailed rewarding the different federal and state requirements that prescriptions, as well as the drugs that exist on them, need to follow. We took a look at how to dispose of your hazardous and non-hazardous substances, what the DEA and FDA have to say about controlled substances, as well as some of the calculations you are advised to know about.

As a pharmacy technician, you will most likely be faced with a few recalls throughout your career. Although your role in these recalls will either be contact tracing or removing the recalled medications from the pharmacy shelves, you will play a pivotal role. But, what is the main reason that recalls are done? To ensure patient safety! Recalls can even be avoided should effective quality assurance processes be implemented. For this reason, our next chapter will focus on "Patient Safety and Quality Assurance."

Chapter Four: Patient Safety and Quality Assurance

This segment of the PTCB exam is one that is very important. Not only does it make up 26.25% of the entire test, but it also provides you with effective mechanisms to ensure patient safety and the quality of the medication you are dispensing. In this chapter, we will be going through medications that look alike and sound alike, types of errors that can occur and how they can be reduced, instances when a pharmacist needs to intervene, as well as important hygiene and cleaning standards.

The Potential of Risk-Inducing Events Occurring

As a pharmacy technician, you will always need to remain focused on your job. Otherwise, instances such as medication errors can occur. Now although there are a lot of steps one can take to ensure these errors do not happen, sometimes the odd error will slip through the cracks. This is why we all need to be mindful of our own personal strategies to combat this. Not only will it save you time, but it will leave you stress-free and error-free!

High Alert/Risk Medications

Medications that fall under this category are those that will most likely cause patient harm if they are taken incorrectly or if they are part of an error. An example of this would be warfarin, a blood-thinning medication that can be life-threatening when present in overdose. The same life-threatening effect can happen if it has a drug interaction with another drug or if a drug-monitoring error were to occur.

Thankfully, there are resources available to identify high-risk medications. The main resource that is used is the Institute for Safe Medication Practices (ISMP) which consists of all the high-alert medications such as warfarin.

Look-Alike/Sound-Alike (LASA) Medications

A big safety concern is giving a patient the wrong medication. However, two of the main causes of this specific medication error are based on two medications that either sound or look alike. Now, as a pharmacy technician, it is important to know that just because two drugs sound or look the same, it does not mean they can be substituted between each other and used interchangeably. It is these errors in drug selection, and even communication with a patient, that can result in life-threatening complications and, in the worst cases, death.

In cases where two drugs look alike, it remains your duty to double-check the chosen drug and its strength, ensuring they correlate with the prescription. A way to manage this is by implementing the "tall man lettering" system.

Implementable Error Prevention Strategies

Before you are a pharmacy technician, you are a human. This means you will make mistakes; it is inevitable. However, any and all healthcare personnel need to be extra vigilant when performing their duties. You should strive never to cause a medication error; however, if it does happen, you need to be able to learn from the situation. Luckily, multiple different practices are instituted to drastically decrease the chances of a medication error occurring and, better yet, prevent it from reaching the patient. Let's go through a few of these practices and strategies.

Giving the Correct Order to the Correct Patient

As a pharmacy technician, you need to try your best to always give the correct order to the correct patient. Typically, the five "rights" govern what you need to adhere to when dispensing medication to a patient. You need to make sure it is the right drug, present at the right dose, with the right time intervals, and given by the right route to the right patient. By solidifying the five rights in your mind, you will drastically decrease the chances of a medication error occurring.

Always make sure the following is checked before handing the patient's order to them:

- Ensure that the patient's name and date of birth are correct before handing the medication to them.
- Confirm their place of residence.
- Mention what they were here to pick up. For example, you can say, "Good morning, Mrs. Y. I have your diabetic tablets and insulin ready. Will that be all for you today?"

Tall Man Lettering

This strategy is used to differentiate LASA medications from each other. An example of these types of medication could be hydralazine, which is an anti-hypertensive drug, and hydroxyzine, a potent antihistamine. To notice the difference between these two drugs, usually the different letters, and in this case, the middle three, will be written with capital letters. In this case, the labels will read hydrALAzine or hydrOXYzine. This is a great way to really eliminate discrepancies and medication errors!

Inventory Separation

Managing inventory is a large part of any pharmacy technician's job. From receiving new products, identifying where the drugs need to be placed, as well as removing expired stock and sending recalled medication to the manufacturers, inventory management, in general, is very laborious!

However, by separating your medications by Schedule and formulation, you are not only able to perform effective inventory checks, but you are also able to identify the general area where a drug will be.

Leading and Trailing Zeros

This concept refers to the recording process as well as when you are writing instructions to a patient on how to take their medication. When you are required to use whole numbers, you do not need to put a trailing zero. For example, if you have five tablets, you would write it as 5 and not 5.0. Also, do not forget the units!

Contrastingly, if you are dealing with a fraction of a whole number, such as when a pediatric patient needs to be given medication, a leading zero is placed before the decimal point to decrease overdose risk. For example, if the child requires 0.75 milliliters of pain medication, the zero will need to be present. Yes, to us, it would be irrational for a child to receive 75 milliliters of liquid, but we are not the general public. So, we need to make it as explicitly clear as possible.

Using Barcodes

Similar to the National Drug Code (NDC) that one would use, barcodes are more effective. Not only are they unique to each pharmaceutical product, but they are used as a secondary check to ensure you have chosen the correct product. This task can be completed through the use of a scanner.

The Use of Abbreviations

As a pharmacy technician, you will most likely need to read abbreviations from prescribing practitioners. However, when you are writing the patient's instructions, do not use abbreviations. Instead of writing QD, make sure to write either "daily" or "once a day." Yes, abbreviations are faster to use; however, writing out the instructions solidifies what you are doing and will prevent errors from occurring.

Issues That Require a Pharmacist's Intervention

As a pharmacy technician, you will not be able to do everything a pharmacist can. Usually, every pharmacy needs to have a pharmacist present at all times to answer any questions or concerns that may occur. Making sure you have a good relationship with your pharmacists will only make you a better pharmacy technician. They have a wealth of information that will require you to call upon them for assistance when posed with a clinical scenario.

It is important to note that a clinical problem should never be tackled solely by a pharmacy technician.

Drug Utilization Reviews (DURs)

In order for a patient to receive their medication as a first issue or refill, a pharmacist needs to conduct a DUR. This involves obtaining a comprehensive summary of all the patient's OTC and prescription medications. The pharmacist will then ensure that there are no specific drug-drug interactions or adverse drug events that can occur. If a patient has a clinical question or you suspect misuse or abuse as the pharmacy technician, the pharmacist is to be contacted and asked to intervene where necessary.

Adverse Drug Events (ADEs)

These events are unwanted and typically result from the normal use of a drug or its potential misuse. An ADE can occur as a result of a medication error or from the actual act of the patient taking the medication. Your adverse events have the potential to cause serious injury and can even be life-threatening. When compared to your "side effects," an adverse event is more serious in nature.

As soon as an adverse event is reported to you, you will need to contact your pharmacist and inform them of the adverse event's origin. Detailed documentation is then filled in on the patient's profile so that the same adverse event does not happen in the future. In terms of ensuring adequate quality assurance, the pharmacist should also report the adverse event via the FDA Adverse Event Reporting System (FAERS).

Over-the-Counter (OTC) Medication Recommendations

OTC medications are those that can be obtained without a prescription. These medications are usually not highly regulated and treat very minor ailments and symptoms. For example, you would most likely go and get some OTC medication for a headache if you have the flu or your nose is so blocked you are struggling to breathe through your nostrils. Medications that fall within the OTC category include acetaminophen (an analgesic), cetirizine (an antihistamine), diphenhydramine (an antihistamine), and phenylephrine (a nasal decongestant).

If a patient comes in and they ask clinical questions regarding OTC medications, the pharmacist should always be available to answer these questions. A pharmacist can also make recommendations on which OTC medications will be of benefit in treating the patient's current ailments.

Therapeutic Substitution

This action, performed primarily by pharmacists, is when a specific medication is switched within its drug class to another medication. The key here is that it is done without first contacting and gaining approval from the prescriber. The therapeutic substitution will usually happen in federal facilities and in hospitals. The reason for this is that these facilities usually only keep very limited types of drugs in the pharmacy.

It is important that we establish the difference between therapeutic substitution and generic substitution. The latter is when you are exchanging the drug's generic version for that of the brand name. For example, if Zoloft has been prescribed to you, sertraline, which is the generic of Zoloft, will be dispensed to the patient.

Misuse of Medication

The misuse of medication is a public health crisis. Whether the misuse was unintentional or intentional, the process in which the misuse occurred could have happened in many different ways. For example, a patient who believes they have depression could've self-medicated by using their cousin's sertraline. Another instance of medication misuse is for patients who suffer from elevated levels of anxiety taking lorazepam more often than what was prescribed to them.

Although the above aspects of misuse are for the process of treating a clinical condition, there are instances where medication is misused and abused for other reasons. For example, some people may misuse oxycodone because they want to "get high." However, it does not matter what the intent of the misuse is, the pharmacy technician and pharmacist need to always be vigilant.

Adherence to Medication

Some patients may find that the reason their conditions are either uncontrolled, or they have not been cured, is that they are not remaining adherent to their medication. The key here is being able to identify the causes of the patient not taking their medication and addressing it promptly.

A pharmacist may need to repetitively counsel a patient on the necessity of them taking their medication. Maybe a patient does not understand why they need to take medication or are sharing their medication with family members, which leads them to not have enough to get them through the month. Non-adherence is multifactorial in nature, and adherence strategies like alarm clocks for patients who just forget to take their medication should be recommended.

Post-Immunization Follow-Up

A pharmacist is able to administer vaccines; however, they always need to ensure that detailed patient information is taken in the event that, post-immunization, an adverse reaction occurs. This is what should be documented:

- The demographics of the patient.
- The prescriber that ordered the vaccine.
- The dose of vaccine that was given.
- The administration route and site.
- The vaccine's expiration date.
- The vaccine's lot number.
- The name of the person who administered the vaccine, including the date of administration.

To close off the information loop, the pharmacist will send a copy of the vaccine administration document to the prescribing practitioner. It is important to also note that an adverse effect may not happen immediately. There have been some reports of these adverse effects occurring up to two weeks after vaccine administration. Should an adverse reaction occur, it is to be reported to the Vaccine Adverse Event Reporting System (VAERS), which is run by both the FDA and the CDC. This reporting is important as it may assist in identifying specific adverse event patterns that occur with a specific vaccine.

Allergies

A pharmacist should ensure that all of a patient's allergies are present on their profile. Not only is this documented before the patient's script is dispensed, but it should always be asked to confirm the system's information. Remember, a patient can have an allergy to both scheduled and OTC medication. A patient should also not have a drug that has caused a reaction rechallenged.

Drug Interactions

As the pharmacist goes ahead and performs a DUR, they will note any potential drug-drug interactions. Should there be a very minor interaction, the pharmacist should ensure that the patient is counseled and that they are given monitoring parameters to identify if they should seek immediate help or not.

However, if the interaction is known to cause life-threatening effects, it is under no circumstances to be dispensed to the patient!

Event Reporting Procedures

Adverse events will occur at some point in your career as a pharmacy technician. It is these events as well as any medication errors that occur, which need to be both internally and externally reported and documented. This will always ensure that all quality assurance practices are upheld!

You also need to know that the reporting of these events and errors is not meant to be punitive in nature. It is done to understand which processes are implemented at the pharmacy and how adaptations can occur to ensure it does not happen again.

Medication Errors

It does not matter which step of the medication-use process a person is at. Medication errors can occur. Ranging from transcribing to prescribing errors, as well as administering and dispensing errors, one can see how many points are present where an error can occur. The main point of an error is to learn from it. A pharmacist needs to be able to identify at what point the error occurred to make sure it does not happen again. As a pharmacy technician, you will be assisting them with this.

If it is found that the medication error happened in the pharmacy, it needs to be internally investigated and documented. The error also needs to be communicated to the prescribing practitioner, as well as the patient. This is not to put the person at fault in the spotlight but more so that the patient is monitored for any unexpected adverse event resulting from the error.

Adverse Effects

ADEs are reported to the FAERS program. If the FDA starts to notice a trend in a particular medication causing a specific ADE, they will meet with the drug's manufacturer to discuss and alter manufacturing processes and/or ingredients to mitigate the issue.

Based on the severity of the ADE and the frequency of it being reported, the FDA may request a black box warning to be placed on the label or, in severe cases, a product recall. Medications with very severe ADEs can be permanently removed from all stores, never to be manufactured again.

Product Integrity

As a pharmacy technician, you will have the opportunity to identify and ensure that all pharmaceutical products being dispensed are safe, efficacious, and according to the standards set by the pharmaceutical manufacturer. As soon as a product is compromised, whether due to an increase in moisture levels, the altering of storage temperatures, or inadequate storage overall, the effect of the drug is compromised.

A product's integrity also starts to become altered as soon as its expiration date is bypassed. An example of this can be seen with melatonin, a medicine used to help treat insomnia. Melatonin can be present in a sublingual dosage form, meaning you place the tablet underneath your tongue. However, if its storage bottle is not properly closed, the tablets will become brittle and ineffective.

MedWatch

A program created by the FDA, MedWatch is the platform whereby both patients and any healthcare practitioner can report any medication that has caused an adverse reaction. This is an entirely electronic process, where the FDA will pick up commonalities and issue a recall of the medication should a problem occur. These electronic forms can be obtained on the FDA website.

Near Miss

Also known as a "close call," a near miss is when a medication error has occurred but is identified and does not reach the patient. In order for all processes to be continuously improved, all near misses need to be internally documented and reported.

Let's solidify this concept by looking at an example. As a pharmacy technician, you are returning all of the uncollected medications back to the shelves. However, you notice that Mr. X's blood pressure medication was in the same bag as Mrs. L's blood-thinning medication. This means that Mrs. L could have erroneously taken Mr. X's blood pressure medication, needing to be recorded as an internal dispensing error. It is because this error did not reach Mrs. L that it is a near miss.

Root Cause Analysis (RCA)

Usually, an RCA is done to understand why a problem occurred in the first place. This means trailing through the entire filling and dispensing process to try and figure out where the error occurred. As a pharmacy technician, you need to understand the origin of the error to ensure that it does not happen again. An example of this could be Mr. G, who picked up his warfarin tablets but noticed they were yellow instead of blue. After doing an RCA, it was found he was given the 2.5 mg tablets instead of the 4 mg tablets. This final check was also not picked up by the pharmacist.

To combat the above scenario, implementing a barcode scanner can not only confirm you are giving the right medication but also ensures that the entire medication selection process is easier and more seamless.

Types of Prescription Errors

Errors on prescriptions are a lot more common than one would think. This is why all pharmacy personnel, especially the pharmacy technician and pharmacist, need to always be vigilant when preparing a prescription for dispensing. Spend some extra time and double-check all of your work! You need to understand your duties, as well as what consequences come of not performing them correctly. Let's jump into a few of the errors one can get on a prescription.

Abnormal Doses

Quality assurance is the responsibility of the pharmacist, making sure that the dose written on the prescription is able to perform its desired therapeutic action. This is why it is important to understand the different types of dosage forms and routes of administration that common medications can occur in. Furthermore, ensuring that knowledge of standard dosing is present will enable quick identification of abnormal doses. If you identify this error, make sure to double-check it with your pharmacist before continuing with the filling process.

For example, morphine comes in a bunch of different concentrations. Let's say you get a prescription that reads: Morphine Sulphate 100 mg/5 ml oral solution, take 5 ml by mouth every 2–4 hours as needed for hospice care, dispense 30 ml. If you take a look at the dosing, even though they are in hospice care, taking this concentration every two hours can result in 1,200 mg/day of morphine. This is a toxic dose of morphine! Thus, when contacted, the prescribing practitioner made an error and meant to write the concentration as 10 mg/5 ml. This makes a lot more sense!

Early Refill

Early refills are easy to identify as a patient's insurance will reject the claim if it is not the exact date when the patient is to collect their medication. Now usually, this isn't a problem for non-controlled drugs. But you may be asking what would happen in the instance where medication has been lost or altered, or the patient needs a greater quantity because they are traveling internationally. Well, there are ways to override the insurance for it to be successfully processed. But if, for some reason, the insurance does not pay for the early refill, the patient does have the option to pay cash for it instead.

With controlled medications, federal and state regulations do not allow early refills. The only exception to this rule would be if the prescriber grants it under certain circumstances. Even though the prescriber has asked for this to occur, there is still a chance that the insurance will reject the claim. Usually, there is a 1–2 day leeway that pharmacies will allow for, especially if the patient is out of medication before their next refill.

Incorrect Quantity

It is important to always ensure the correct quantity of medications is dispensed to a patient. Not only does this assist with continuity of care, but it also streamlines the patient's healthcare journey. Legally, you are able to dispense less than what is found on a prescription. But, it is illegal to dispense more! So, if you were faced with a patient who has a prescription for 84 days of a non-controlled medication, and they only ask for 28 days of medication, you are legally allowed to do so. The remaining quantity will be documented on the patient's profile for when they would come and refill their medication.

Some prescribing practitioners may put "QS" on their scripts. This then gives the pharmacy technician and the pharmacist liberty to provide the quantity sufficient for the treatment period the prescriber has written down.

Incorrect Patient

Not everyone has unique names and surnames. Thus, the chances of there being more than one patient with the same name, surname, or both, are very high! A way to deduce incorrect patient errors is by asking the patient their date of birth and then correlating that with the profiles in front of you. In the unlikely case, when the date of birth is the same, you can then look at the street address.

There have even been cases where parents will give their children the same name as them. In these cases, you can look at the suffix or title of the patient. Usually, you can tell the difference based on the suffixes Jr. and Sr. (junior and senior).

Incorrect Drug

You can choose the incorrect drug when going to the shelves to pick up the medication for the order or through the data entry process. Remember we spoke about LASA medications? Well, this could be the result, or it could just be pure negligence. An example of this would be Dexilant, a Proton Pump Inhibitor (PPI) available in 30 mg and 60 mg. Duloxetine, used to treat depression, also has these strengths. If you don't pay attention and mix these two up, you may find yourself giving a patient an anti-depressant instead of helping treat their heartburn.

Calculations You Should Know

You receive the following prescription: Prednisolone 15 mg/5 ml oral solution, take 45 mg by mouth once daily for 5 days, quantity to dispense is QS. What would the dose be per day in milliliters, and how many milliliters would need to be dispensed to fulfill the prescription? This is how we are going to tackle this problem:

- The concentration of prednisolone is 15 mg/5 ml, which equates to 3 mg/1 ml.
- If the patient needs 45 mg per dose, we can divide that by 3 mg to get the amount of millimeters needed per dose. In this case, it is 15 milliliters.
- With the 15 milliliters being given once a day, multiplying it by the 5 days, you will get an answer of 75 milliliters. This is the total amount you will need to dispense to fulfill all the script's requirements.

Hygiene and Cleaning Standards

Because we all work in the medical field, we have the opportunity to spread illnesses and infections to other coworkers and members of the general public.

This even goes as far as us infecting medications that, when ingested by patients, cause them to become ill. Especially for this reason, everyone needs to practice good and proper personal hygiene! This will result in a decrease in the possibility of infecting patients and contaminating medications.

Standards also included in this overarching theme include staying at home when you are ill, as well as ensuring all surfaces and equipment are clean before being used again. Let's take a look at some of the hygiene and cleaning standards you should be aware of.

Handwashing

This is probably the easiest and simplest way to implement infection control. Make sure you wash your hands before and after any compounding procedure or process that needs you to be in direct contact with any drug product. This even includes making sure to wash your hands before donning your PPE!

Personal Protective Equipment (PPE)

PPE is required for any and all types of compounding procedures. When getting ready to don your PPE, you will need to make sure that the correct process is followed. You will usually work from the "dirtiest" to the "cleanest" segments of your PPE. This is done to reduce the possibility of any contamination occurring. Below is the general order you can follow when donning your PPE:

- Make sure you have removed all of your excess outer garments and do not have any makeup, piercings, or jewelry on your body.
- Cover your shoes and hair with the relevant covers. This also includes any facial hair.
- You can then choose to either wear a face shield or a face mask.
- Using the appropriate handwashing technique, wash your hands.
- Put on your compounding-specific gown.
- You can now put on your sterile gloves. Should you be moving between different drug products, make sure to sterilize your hands with alcohol before touching the other drug product.

Counting Trays

All of the spatulas and counting trays that you use need to be cleaned both before and after they are used. You can make use of 70% isopropyl alcohol to assist in reducing the risk of contamination. It is also important that, as a pharmacy technician, you are aware of the different counting trays that are used purely for penicillin and drugs that contain sulfur. This is of vital importance as a speck present in a patient who is allergic to the medication can result in life-threatening effects.

Countertop

All pharmacy countertops need to be regularly wiped down throughout the day. To decrease contamination, as well as ensure that bacterial growth does not occur, you can make use of isopropyl alcohol or another suitable detergent.

Equipment

Cleanliness needs to always be maintained in a pharmacy, no matter what your hours of operation are. Make sure that you are cleaning the following equipment, areas, and surfaces at least once a day:

- Make sure to dust the storage areas that contain all of the pharmacy's equipment and medication.
- Wipe down all tools and equipment needed for the preparation and dispensing of medication. This includes, but is not limited to, keyboards, working surfaces, phones and telephones, and computer screens.
- Ensure all the floors are either mopped or vacuumed.
- Make sure the pharmacy work area is free from trash.
- In settings where a patient area is present, make sure to clean it as well.

Equipment that is used during the compounding process, such as your mortar and pestle, scales, and Erlenmeyer flasks, should also be cleaned regularly. This also includes cleaning them if they have not been used for a long period of time. You would not want there to be any dust in your final product!

One can only imagine how important patient safety is. After all, they are putting their lives and trust in our hands to make them feel better. This works hand in hand with quality assurance and ensuring that all medication that patients receive is of the highest quality.

In this chapter, we focused on areas where errors are more common, taking a look at high-risk medications and a part of the LASA category. We delved into strategies that can be implemented to prevent errors, as well as situations where pharmacy technicians will need the pharmacist to intervene. Other than focusing on when different kinds of prescription errors can occur, should an error still occur, we went through what the process is for reporting these events. Lastly, we all know that hygiene and cleanliness are important, both personally and professionally. So, we reiterated a few of the main hygiene standards that need to be remembered.

You have now tackled and completed three of the four knowledge domains for the PTCB exam. You are almost there! You've successfully dealt with everything that is patient- and medication-related. All that is left for you to delve into is the fourth knowledge domain—Order Entry and Processing.

Chapter Five: Order Entry and Processing

Questions that pertain to Order Entry and Processing will constitute 21.25% of your PTCB exam. This is also another fun section, as you delve into understanding how to perform non-sterile compounding, which calculations you need to be able to do, equipment that you will need to administer drugs, a further explanation on expiration dates, and an understanding of National Drug Code (NDC) numbers. It is in this section that you will also be taught how to identify and understand the symbols that are present on a prescription.

Non-Sterile Compounding

Standards are present that classify compounding as either non-sterile or sterile. These standards can be found in the USP 795 regulations. These regulations inform us that non-sterile compounding includes the need to wear the proper PPE and ensure that before you begin compounding, all services are clean. There is such a large diversity of things that can be compounded, but here are some general steps to take into consideration:

- Create a formula based on the prescription. This way, you will be able to see how much of each ingredient you will need.
- Put on the required PPE, and make sure to wash your hands.
- If you need any hardware supplies, make sure to get them before starting to compound. These can include your graduated cylinders or any scales you may need.

- Using measuring tools, weigh out all of the ingredients.
- Combine the ingredients as per a specific recipe, ensuring that the order and ratios of all constituents are correct.
- Make a written note of how much of each ingredient was used.
- Make sure there is a label present on the final product, which includes what the final strengths of the ingredients are.

Ointments

Ointments are typically used as topical preparations with the main goal of treating dermatological conditions (i.e., conditions affecting the skin). There are instances where ointments can be used on/in other parts of the body, such as in the eyes, as ophthalmic ointments. An example of an ophthalmic ointment is erythromycin.

The makeup of an ointment is predominantly oil-based and can also be termed "water in oil" preparations. Your ointments differ from creams as the latter is more water-based and is referred to as "oil in water" preparations. Whether you are preparing an ointment or cream, you will use the spatulation process. This process enables the mixing of powders and other semi-solids onto an oiled slab. When mixing, make sure you are using a geometric method (i.e., adding small bits of the ingredients at a time).

The storage of your ointment, once compounded, can either be in a tube or a jar.

Mixtures

A mixture is seen as a variety of formulations. It is also not limited to a single active or inactive ingredient. It contains numerous ingredients, all of the different types, in order to create a compound. The process of simple mixing is one where you can combine a solid with a liquid, two different solids, or two different liquids together.

Mixtures also need to be created geometrically. For example, the magic mouthwash that can be used to treat both mucositis and mouth pain uses a 1:1:1 ratio of diphenhydramine, a liquid antacid, as well as 2% of viscous lidocaine. So, seeing as all of these ingredients are uniform in nature, if you were to create 300 ml of this mixture, you would need to add 100 ml of each ingredient based on the ratio.

A type of liquid mixture is that of a suspension. This mixture is where you have powdered medication that is combined with liquid, usually sterile water. It is because suspensions can have an unpleasant taste that flavoring agents can enhance.

Liquids

A liquid consists of two segments, namely a solute and a solvent. A solute is a part that is the active pharmaceutical ingredient and is dissolved in the solvent. One of the most important aspects of a liquid to remember is that you need to ensure that your solute is evenly distributed throughout the solvent, i.e., your liquid needs to be homogenous!

Seeing as suspensions are also classified as being a liquid, you will need to redistribute their contents before every use. This is easily done by shaking the preparation sufficiently, allowing any particles that settled at the bottom of the bottle to be reconstituted.

Emulsions

An emulsion occurs when two liquids are unable to be mixed together (i.e., they are immiscible). An emulsion will consist of a liquid that will be dispersed (known as the discontinuous phase) through the entirety of another liquid (known as the continuous phase).

An example of an emulsion is an oil in water preparation. We know that water and oil do not mix together. Thus, to disperse the oil throughout the water, one would need to shake the bottle vigorously. Creams and ointment or lotion bases are prime examples of topical formulations, which are emulsions.

Suppositories

A solid formulation, suppositories are administered rectally but, in some cases, can be inserted vaginally. A suppository consists of your active pharmaceutical ingredient that is suspended in a particular base. One of the most common bases is cocoa butter. Because suppositories placed rectally bypass first-pass metabolism, they have the ability to treat both systemic and localized conditions. The storage of suppositories is usually in a thick foil wrapper. This is because suppositories will melt at body temperature.

There are three main manners in which suppositories can be prepared. These are compression molding, hand rolling, and fusion molding. The simplest of these is the hand-rolling technique which is literally mixing the active ingredient in the suppository's base and manipulating it into a uniform cone shape. Suppositories are perfect dosage forms to give to patients who are unable to take medication orally or, more specifically, to those who have issues with their bowels.

Enemas

An enema is a type of preparation that treats ulcerative colitis, constipation, IBS, and a bunch of other bowel-related conditions. Enemas will also be used to clean out the bowels before a patient undergoes surgery. However, although they work very well, very few individuals know how they actually work. An enema is not systemically absorbed. Rather, it interacts with the lining of your colon, causing overwhelming peristalsis and removal of the contents of your bowel. They work very rapidly, so care should be taken when administering an enema. Please be sure you are near a toilet if you need to use an enema!

Necessary Calculations for Non-Sterile Compounding

Non-sterile compounding requires an aptness for mathematics. More specifically, you will need to know how much of each ingredient you will need to add in order to derive the required strength. However, many prescribers enjoy using percentage strengths which can become very confusing depending on the preparation. There are three percentage strengths you should be aware of. They are as follows:

- Weight/Weight (w/w%): This percentage strength refers to the amount of grams of an ingredient you will find in 100 grams of the product.
- Volume/Volume (v/v%): This percentage strength refers to the amount of milliliters of an ingredient you will find in 100 milliliters of the final product.
- Weight/Volume (w/v%): This percentage strength refers to the amount of grams of an ingredient you will find in 100 milliliters of the final product.

Vocabulary and Procedures

Within the pharmacy domain, there is a certain degree of jargon you will need to understand as a pharmacy technician. It is by understanding the nuances behind all of the calculations, procedures, and work-related jargon that you are building yourself up to become the most competent pharmacy technician! The more confident you become in these aspects, the better you will be able to communicate with others, promote patient care, and succeed in your daily duties and tasks.

Some More Calculations

You've dealt with a few of the more common calculations up until this point. However, now we are going to focus on a few of the more specific types of calculations. Arithmetic is important and will be used daily as a pharmacy technician. Most of the calculations you'll be able to do in your head; however, if you are uncertain, use a calculator. Luckily, you have a pharmacist who will check all your work and calculations before dispensing the prescription to the patient! So, what types of calculations will we be going through?

Formulas

A specific method under this subset is known as dimensional analysis. This refers to calculating the "wanted quantity" by using ratios. The general rule of thumb here is to use the following:

$$\text{Given QT x CF} = \text{Wanted QT}$$

With the above equation, your QT refers to quantity, and your CF is the Conversion Factor. By solidifying this into an example, we can ask ourselves how we would convert 20 inches into centimeters. We would do this as follows:

- We know that one inch is equal to 2.54 cm.
- Thus when we multiply 20 by the conversion factor of 2.54 cm, we get the "Wanted QT."
- The answer to this conversion would be 50.8 cm.

In some problems, you may actually need more than one Conversion Factor. For example, if you are faced with a scenario where a male patient who weighs 141 pounds needs 5 mg/kg per day of a specific medication, how would you go about calculating his total daily prescription in mg? Well, you would tackle this problem as follows:

- Your first step is converting pounds to kilograms. This is done by identifying that one kilogram is equal to 2.2 pounds. Thus, to obtain an x value, you would have 1 kilogram as the numerator and 2.2 pounds as the denominator. Remember, when you move a value from one side of an equal side to the other, it becomes the denominator.
- So, taking 141 pounds and multiplying it by (1 kg/2.2 lb) will give you the total amount of kilograms of your patient. This number is 64.09 kg.
- Now by multiplying 64.09 kg by 5 mg, you will be able to calculate his total daily dose based on the rationale that he needs 5 mg for every kg of bodyweight.
- Thus 64.09 kg multiplied by 5 will give you a total daily dose of 320.45 mg.

Ratios and Proportions

A ratio is seen as the relative value that will exist between two numbers. It can be the conversion of a fraction, which, when large enough, can be simplified to give us a basic understanding of the ratio of one substance to the next. For example, a fraction of ½ can be represented as a ratio of 1:2. Seemingly, a fraction of 4/8 can be represented as a ratio of 4:8, which, when simplified, will also give a ratio of 1:2. Remember, it is not ever only two ingredients that can have a ratio. Remember when we discussed the magic mouthwash? That was a 1:1:1 ratio of all three of its ingredients.

But then, what is a proportion? A proportion is a relationship that exists between two ratios. These can be expressed as follows:

- a:b = c:d
- a/b = c/d
- a:b:: c:d

As you use the above values and fill in the required values, you can use the proportions blueprints to calculate a missing value. For example, if you have a prescription which mentions a concentration of 100 mg of morphine in every 5 ml, how would you go about dispensing the required amount of ml that equates to only 10 mg of morphine? Well, you would do this as follows:

- You know that 100 mg = 5 ml. These will be your numerators.
- You know that you want 10 mg, so this will be your denominator on the mg side.
- You are looking for the denominator on the milliliter side to see how many milliliters are needed to contain 10 mg of morphine. Let's call that "x."
- So, you will then have 100 mg/10 mg = 5 ml/x.
- Through cross-multiplication, you will end with 100 x = 50 ml.
- This is then expressed as x = 50 ml/100.
- The answer is then 0.5 ml.

Allegations

The allegation method enables you as a pharmacy technician to create a concentration of a specific solution using two different solutions that have the same ingredients but exist at different strengths. For you to create your desired concentration, you will need to have a solution that has a concentration higher than, and a contraction that is lower than your desired concentration.

It is by calculating the difference in the percentage strengths that you can identify the number of parts, as well as the volume of each part needed to provide you with the volume of your desired end product.

The higher percentage solution will be labeled A, your lower percentage solution will be labeled B, your desired percentage of your final product will be C, the amount of parts of your higher percentage solution will be D, and the amount of parts of your lower percentage solution will be E. So with this in mind, you will need to factor in the following:

- To calculate D, you will need to take C minus B.
- To calculate E, you will need to take A minus C.
- Then you add D and E together to get the total number of parts needed.
- The final volume of your desired product is then divided by the total amount of parts needed. You will then get a ml/part value.
- You then multiply this ml/part value by D and E to see how much ml of each solution you will need!

Let's solidify this concept through the use of an example. If you were posed with the following question: How many milliliters of a 60% solution (A), as well as a 25% solution (B), would you need to create 700 milliliters of a 30% solution (C)? You would tackle this as follows:

- First, calculate D by taking 30% - 25% = 5 parts of your higher percentage solution.
- Secondly, calculate E by taking 60% - 30% = 30 parts of your lower percentage solution.
- By adding the total parts of each together, you are working with 35 parts.
- With your total amount wanted to be 700 ml, you are going to divide it by 35 to get the amount of ml/part. This value is 20 ml/part.
- Multiplying 20 ml by D will give you the amount of the higher percentage solution you will need, which in this case is 100 ml of the 60% solution.
- Multiplying 20 ml by E will give you the amount of the lower percentage solution you will need, which in this case is 600 ml of the 25% solution.

- Add the two quantities together, and you will get your desired 700 ml of a 30% solution.

Conversions

There are multiple different types of conversions you need to know as a pharmacy technician. This is because you will be interacting with prescribing practitioners who will all use different units of measurement. Learning all about the different kinds of conversions will also enable you to provide your patient with the easiest way to take their medication. Instead of telling them to take 30 ml, you can tell them to take 2 tablespoons. The conversions will be divided into those that are volume-based, weight-based, and length-based. The volume-based conversions you should know are:

- One teaspoon (tsp) = 5 ml
- One tablespoon (tbsp) = 15 ml
- One liter (L) = 10 deciliters (dL) = 100 centiliters (cL) = 1,000 milliliters (ml) = 1,000,000 microliters (mcL)
- One milliliter (ml) = approximately 20 drops
- One gallon (gal) = 4 quarts (qts)
- One fluid ounce (fl oz) = 29.6 milliliters (ml)
- One quart (qt) = 2 pints
- One pint (pt) = approximately 473 milliliters (ml)

Your weight-based conversions you should know are:

- One kilogram (kg) = 2.2 pounds (lb)
- One gram (g) = 10 decigrams (dg) = 100 centigrams (cg) = 1,000 milligrams (mg) = 1,000,000 micrograms (mcg)
- One grain = 64.8 milligrams (mg)
- One pound (lb) = 16 ounces (oz)
- One pound (lb) = approximately 454 grams (g)

The length-based conversion that you should know is:

- One inch = 2.54 centimeters (cm)

So, to put all of this into perspective, let's look at an example. You have a patient who was given a specific eye drop with the following directions: Place 1 drop in each eye 6 times per day for 7 days. The quantity needed to be supplied is QS. The question is now how much you would need to dispense in order to cover the patient's entire course of therapy. The eye drops are only available in 2.5 ml, 5 ml, and 10 ml containers. This can be calculated as follows:

- We know that the total amount of drops for the entire course is 84 drops.
- We also know that there are approximately 20 drops per 1 milliliter.
- When we divide the 84 drops by 20, we get an equivalent of 4.2 ml.
- With the closest container being 5 ml, that will be the best selection for this patient.

Sig Codes

Sig codes are relatively easy to understand because all they really do is tell us how the prescribing practitioner wants the patient to take their medication. As a pharmacy technician, you are the middleman between what you see on the prescription and what is present on the patient's label. Ultimately, sig codes are abbreviations that are on a prescription.

So let's jump right into some of the different sig codes you will come across. We will focus on the sig codes for frequency and route of administration. The sig codes for frequency are:

- QD = Once daily
- QOD = Every other day
- QOW = Every other week
- BID = Twice a day
- TID = Three times a day
- QID = Four times a day
- Q4H = Every 4 hours
- Q6H = Every 6 hours
- Q8H = Every 8 hours
- Q12H = Every 12 hours

These are the most common sig codes for describing the route of administration the drug in question should be administered:

- PO = By mouth
- SL = Sublingual (placed under the tongue)
- BUCC = Buccally (placed inside the cheek)
- TOP = Topically (placed on the skin)
- SC or SUBQ = Subcutaneously
- IM = Intramuscularly
- IN = Intranasally
- IV = Intravenously
- ID = Intradermally
- IT = Intrathecally
- INH = Inhale
- PV = Per vagina or vaginally
- PR = Per rectum or rectally
- Opth = Ophthalmic (i.e., eye)
- Otic = Ear

These are the most common sig codes you will need to know to pass your PTCB Exam. Know these off by heart as they will not only help you in the exam but also in your professional career as a pharmacy technician.

Roman Numerals

Now although these aren't used as commonly within the pharmacy domain, there are still those practitioners or healthcare professionals who will make use of them. So, to avoid any issues, we are going to tell you the basics of roman numerals. The most common number values for each roman numeral are as follows:

- SS = ½
- I (i) = One
- II (ii) = Two
- III (iii) = Three
- IV (iv) = Four
- V (v) = Five

- X (x) = Ten
- L = 50
- C = 100
- D = 500
- M = 1,000

It is important to note that when placed together in ascending format, the letters are added together. However, if you notice a smaller value before a larger value, subtraction from the larger value needs to occur. For example, if you look at IV, it is the number 4, whereas VI will be the number 6. The same concept applies to XLI, which equals 41, whereas LXI will equal 61.

Medical Terminology

Within the healthcare system, you can imagine that a lot of medical terminologies are used. Whether you are consulting a prescriber to change a medication that is out of stock or following up on a patient in the hospital, the terminology and verbiage used is a golden thread through the healthcare domain. However, as a pharmacy technician, you are going to need to know a few more specific terms. But do not fret; you will learn a lot of the medical terminology for diagnoses the more you immerse yourself in the field.

By making sure you know the medical terminology, you can close the information loop, put a clinical diagnosis to a patient, and link the medication they are taking with that condition. You will learn that hypertension means high blood pressure and that hyperlipidemia means the patient has high cholesterol levels. There is a smorgasbord of different terminology you will learn. But, all in good time!

Abbreviations

Much like your sig codes, the healthcare sector loves using abbreviations. In most cases, these are standard worldwide; however, there are a few that are used in the United States but not in other parts of the world. Now although this allows for more effective communication, you still need to know what is being said.

To help you along, here is a list of the most common abbreviations used in the clinical domain:

- Stat = Immediately
- PRN = As needed
- Tab = Tablet
- Cap = Capsule
- AAA = Apply to affected area
- Amp = Ampule
- Gtt = Drop
- OS = Left eye
- OD = Right eye
- OU = Both eyes
- AS = Left ear
- AD = Right ear
- AU = Both ears
- AM = Morning
- PM = Evening
- HS = Bedtime
- Q = Every
- UD = As directed
- C = With
- AC = Before meals
- PC = After meals
- NPO = Nil per os (i.e., nothing by mouth)
- Preop = Before surgery
- Postop = After surgery
- N/S = Normal saline
- Oint or ung = Ointment
- Sol = Solution
- Sup = Suppository
- Susp = Suspension
- Syr = Syrup
- Inj = Injection
- TDS = Transdermal delivery system
- ODT = Oral disintegrating tablet
- MDI = Metered dose inhaler

- Neb = Nebulization
- ATC = Around the clock
- NR = No refill
- DAW = Dispense as written
- D/C = Discontinue
- Diag = Diagnosis
- Disp = Dispense
- D5W = Dextrose 5% in water

You can combine the above list with the abbreviations for your conversion measurements discussed earlier in this chapter. If you want to go even more in depth and study a few more abbreviations, you can do a simple Google search to obtain a more extensive list. But, these that have been listed are the ones that will be asked in your PTCB exam.

Other Symbols

Now although the above are the more common abbreviations and sig codes you will use in healthcare, there are a few pharmacy-specific ones you can expect to come across. Let's analyze them based on category.

Days' Supply

Now we know that DS usually stands for "days' supply." But sometimes you may come across a prescription that says "x7D," which means for 7 days. Or you may find "x3Mon," which means for 3 months or "until gone." The latter refers to the time when all of your medication has been used up. Remember, your Schedule III to V medications can be given a supply of up to 90 days. So, saying "until gone" refers to the lapsing of the 90-day period.

Quantity

Some prescribers may represent this by using a number followed by a "#." For example, if they write "#30," it means that 30 tablets need to be dispensed. It is important that you don't confuse this with the "days' supply." Yes, it may make sense if the patient needs to take 1 tablet per day. However, if that is not the case, it could prove to be quite an issue.

You also need to take into consideration the type of preparation the prescriber wants the patient to receive. If it is a liquid, then you'll find the total in milliliters. If it is an ointment, the total will most likely be in grams. Another extra symbol you know by now is "QS," which stands for "quantity sufficient."

Dose

Doses will usually use the conversion units of measurement that we've discussed at the beginning of this chapter. Alternatively, you could find that more specific dosing, such as 2 ml or 3 ml, may be required. In the latter case, patients must be given a syringe and taught how to read off the calibration measurements.

Concentration

Depending on the prescription you have received, the concentration can be expressed in a number of different ways. For instance, you could have commercially known and available concentrations that are standard, such as morphine at 10 mg/5 ml. Or, you could find that a more concentrated solution of morphine exists as 100 mg/5 ml. This is why it is always important to ensure you are giving the patient the correct concentration of the drug.

In cases where you are required to dispense an ointment or cream, they can be represented as a percentage concentration. For example, an eye ointment that contains erythromycin can have a concentration of 0.5%. This can be further represented as a concentration of 5 mg/g. A few more examples of commercially available products are your antibiotics, where amoxicillin oral suspension is present as 400 mg/5 ml, and your azithromycin oral suspension is present as 200 mg/5 ml.

Dilutions

This can be a bit of a new concept, but it is also an important concept you need to fully understand. When you perform a dilution, you are, in essence, decreasing the concentration of the solute that is present in the solution. There is a specific formula that one uses, and it is as follows:

$$Concentration~(1)~X~Quantity~(1) = Concentration~(2)~X~Quantity~(2)$$

The "1" refers to the values of the first liquid, whereas the "2" refers to the values of the second liquid. Let's use an example to solidify the concept. You are asked to dilute lidocaine 5% to create a total of 1,000 ml of lidocaine 2%. How much lidocaine 5% will you need to use to achieve this? Well, let's tackle it as follows:

- You know the concentration (2) and quantity (2), as that is the concentration and quantity you are required to make.
- You also have a concentration (1) as the lidocaine 5%.
- So, if you make quantity (1) represented by "x" and solve for it, you will find that you need 400 ml of lidocaine 5%.
- But you are not done, as you need a total of 1,000 ml. And to get this, you will need to add 600 ml of a specific solvent to achieve the desired quantity and concentration.

Equipment and Supplies Required for Drug Administration

In some cases, simply just using an inhaler doesn't allow for the maximum amount of the drug per dose to enter your body. We can think of it logically. Imagine trying to coordinate the breathing of a three-year-old child who has been diagnosed with asthma. You are asking for an impossibility. So, to make your life easier and to enable a drug to be administered more effectively and accurately, equipment and supplies were created to assist the patient! We are now going to discuss some of the equipment and supplies that are used.

Package Size

Some manufacturers have created a specific "unit-of-use" bottle that allows for heightened stability, especially if the drug is photosensitive and reacts poorly to moisture. An example of this is Aggrenox which is in a unit-of-use bottle with a 60 count and is not under any circumstances to be repackaged. Another example is nitroglycerin which always needs to be in an amber vial due to its photosensitivity.

Under no circumstances should drugs that are photosensitive or react poorly to moisture be left out in the open. This will compromise its efficacy and can result in untoward adverse reactions or a sub-therapeutic effect.

Unit Dose

If you are a pharmacy technician who is working in the hospital, you may find that inpatients are dosed using small, single packages. Not only does this help the ease of administration, but because an inpatient's stay in the hospital is usually rather short, it saves the effort of needing to give them more doses of medication than they actually need.

If you are in a community pharmacy setting, also known as a retail pharmacy, you can give the patient the option to either receive their medication in a blister pack or pouch. If we are able to provide the patient with what they request, their compliance with their medication drastically improves. This is perfect for patients who are cared for by caregivers and cannot fill their own pill boxes.

Diabetic Supplies

These supplies can include insulin pens that are prefilled and calibrated in such a way that a patient is able to administer their own insulin. Given subcutaneously, patients need to be educated on how to load their insulin pen to inject the correct amount of insulin each time. A pen needle is screwed onto the bottom of the prefilled syringe, and after use, only discard the pen needle!

Patients who prefer insulin syringes and drawing their insulin out of a vial will need to be educated on how to understand the unit-to-ml ratio on the syringe. There are even some patients who will have an insulin pump fitted, allowing for short-acting insulin to be administered at a rate that is specific to the patient's needs. These pumps are the perfect invention for those who have their diabetes under control and can effectively make healthy decisions regarding their food.

Diabetics who use a glucose meter (also known as a glucometer) to test their blood sugar levels will require the device, test strips specific for the model of the device, as well as single-use lancets to draw a small amount of blood from their finger. It is important to educate the patients to test their blood sugar before meals!

Spacers

Many individuals, especially the young and elderly, struggle to coordinate their breaths with their inhalers. This led to the invention of a spacer that is attached to the end of the inhaler. A spacer is a chamber that is present between the patient's mouth and the inhaler. It allows for a holding area for the medication once the inhaler is pushed. Patients can then breathe multiple times, increasing the amount of drug that enters the patient's body. A spacer can also be used for patients who struggle with the technique of using an inhaler.

Oral and Injectable Syringes

The three parts that make up an injectable syringe are the plunger, barrel, and needle. Typically, you will push the plunger down, forcing the medication through the barrel and through the tip of the needle. When a new syringe is opened, the barrel is sterile, and when getting ready to draw up your drug from a vial, it should not be manipulated at all. Remember, as soon as you are done administering the injection, discard your contents in a sharps container.

A syringe is calibrated and comes in a variety of different sizes. You always want to make sure you use a syringe that is larger than the total you need to administer. For instance, if you need to prepare 1 ml of cyanocobalamin for your pharmacist to administer, your choice of syringe would be a 3 ml one. Yes, 1 ml syringes exist; however, pulling the plunger out to its maximum to accommodate the 1 ml increases the chances of contaminating the contents of the barrel.

You even get oral syringes that don't have a needle attached. Usually, you would use an oral syringe to administer syrups to children, infants, and hospice patients.

Important Numbers You Need to Know

No, we are not referring to telephone numbers you need to stick on your fridge. We are talking about knowing the expiration dates, lot numbers, and the National Drug Code (NDC) for different drugs. Let's discuss each of these individually.

Lot Numbers

Also known as "batch numbers," these are unique numbers that are given to a specific batch during the process of them getting manufactured. The lot number is usually very effective when there is a recall of a specific drug. You can then trace the lot number, usually imprinted on the box or container of your drug, and know exactly which drugs need to be removed from the shelves and sent back to the manufacturer.

Expiration Dates

Every manufacturer will make sure there is an expiration date on the medication's packaging. In cases where pharmacies repackage drugs or count out from a bulk container to provide the patient with the exact amount of medication, the expiration date is one year from when the medication was counted out. However, if the expiration date given by the manufacturer comes first, that is the date that needs to be adhered to.

National Drug Code (NDC) Numbers

NDC numbers are 10-digit numbers that are present in three segments. The first segment tells you who the manufacturer is, the second the product, and the third the package size the drug is present in. More specifically, the second segment will also give you detailed information about the drug's strength, dosage form, and formulation it is in.

What You Need to Know about Returning Medications And Supplies

One of your main roles as a pharmacy technician will be managing inventory. You will be in charge of maintaining medication stock levels and ensuring all the required supplies are always readily available. But, in some cases, you may need to return some medication or supplies. Knowing where to return them will allow you to seamlessly communicate with them to maybe get some credit for the pharmacy instead of losing time and resulting in a possible complete loss due to expired medications.

Identifying Medications to Return

Some medications are slow movers, meaning that if you order too many, there is a chance they may expire. If you can identify they are soon to expire, you can send them back to the manufacturer for some credit! But how do you actually order enough to prevent this? Well, in most pharmacies, you can print a specific medicine's usage data. Here, you will be able to see how many boxes or containers of a specific medication you sold during that month or year. You can then use this to inform you how many your next order should include.

To ensure you are up to date with which medications are near expiry, constant shelf checks should be conducted. For those medications that move at a low to medium pace, they should be checked every three to six months. For those that are fast movers, a shelf check should be done every two weeks. Over and above these checks, every month, temporary stickers should be placed on those medications that are nearing expiration.

Remember, to qualify for some credit, the medicine should not already have expired!

Dispensable versus Non-dispensable Medications and Supplies

Your dispensable medications are typically those that are great candidates to be returned to the manufacturer for credit. These medications are unopened, are still in mint condition, and are still a good few months from their intended expiration date. The reason they are referred to as being "dispensable" is that they can be redistributed to other pharmacies to be sold. But, this process can only be mediated by the drug's manufacturer.

Your non-dispensable medications are those that are not eligible for credit and that cannot be dispensed to a patient. Examples of these types of medications are those that have had their protective seals tampered with, have evidence of opening, or have already passed their expiration date.

Expired Medications

Now although expired medication cannot be sent to the manufacturer or wholesaler for credit, they still need to be sent to them! The reason for this is that the manufacturer will implement practices to ensure the proper disposal of expired medication. Usually, this is done by incineration; however, in a previous chapter, we've discussed some of the other ways disposal can occur.

Destinations of Return

As soon as a medication qualifies to be returned, depending on the type of medication or supplies it is, it may end up at a very specific destination. When you return medication, it can either be done as a credit return, a "return to stock" order, or via reverse distribution. With there being so many different destinations, let's run through the most common of them.

Credit Return

As previously mentioned, a drug can only be returned for credit if it is unopened, has not been tampered with, and is in good condition. But what defines "good condition?" Well, it means that there is no residue from the patient label or any other prominent markings present on the box. Not to mention that the date it is returned needs to be a good few months before the expiration date on the box.

When sending the medication back to the wholesaler, they will usually charge a 10% to 20% restocking fee that is based on the precalculated return value of the returned products.

Return to Stock

This concept refers to putting already packaged medication back on the shelf should the patient not have come to collect their medication within a two-week period. Because the medication did not leave the pharmacy premises, it can be used to fill a prescription brought in by another patient.

As a pharmacy technician, it is important to remember that as soon as the medication leaves the pharmacy premises, it cannot be returned to stock. The only option is for the patient to hand it in for either disposal or return to the manufacturer of the drug.

Reverse Distribution

This process is when the pharmacy decides to send all of the outdated and unusable drugs back to the drug manufacturer. This is usually for either processing or disposal. But, it is also possible for the medication to be sent to another authorized wholesaler. The key thing to remember is that the medication needs to be unusable and be for the pure intention of disposal. Usually, reverse distribution will occur when a patient does not know what to do with their expired medication and brings it back to the pharmacy.

You have now completed all the information within the fourth knowledge domain! During this chapter, we have focused rather heavily on the procedures that need to be followed when compounding non-sterile products.

We used a lot of calculations and formulas, which we highly advise you to go and reread before taking your exam. We even taught you a new language through sig codes, abbreviations, and some of the more common medical terminology you will come across. The chapter then concluded with us discussing what procedures and steps you need to take to return dispensable, non-dispensable, or expired medication.

You did it! You have now gone through all four knowledge domains that will be tested in the PTCB exam. Now you are ready to try your hand at the practice questions. If you get stuck, use deductive reasoning and check the memorandum at the end of the practice test to see if you were correct. If not, there is an explanation of the correct answer and some tips on how to derive it. What are you waiting for? Set your timer, and go for it!

Chapter Six: Full-Length Practice Test #1

Questions

1. You have a patient who has an infection. She has been prescribed azithromycin. But, she has difficulty swallowing. Which dosage form would be best for her?

    A. A liquid
    B. Use of a nebulizer
    C. A nasogastric tube
    D. An injection

2. As a pharmacy technician, you'll be tasked with compounding ophthalmic preparations. Which dosage form below is typically used for ophthalmic preparations?

    A. An emulsion
    B. An ointment
    C. An elixir
    D. A suppository

3. Best practice is always bringing stock from the back of the shelf to the front when restocking. This ensures that those products with a closer expiration are used first. What is this known as?

    A. Ensuring inventory turnover
    B. Stock rotation
    C. FEFO
    D. Forward expiry stocking

4. Your patient is prescribed the following: Hepatin 25,000 units placed in 250cc of D5W and is to run at 1,000 units/hour. You decide to use a micro-drip set of 60 gtt/ml. What rate should you set it at?

    A. 30 gtt/min
    B. 60 gtt/min
    C. 10 gtt/min
    D. 15 gtt/min

5. What is Ultram ER's generic name?

    A. Morphine
    B. Tramadol Hydrochloride
    C. Codeine
    D. Fentanyl

6. For a drug that needs to be stored at 2 to 8 degrees Celsius, where would the best place be to store it?

    A. The pharmacy's separate freezer
    B. A pharmacy refrigerator for medication
    C. The normal stock shelves
    D. In its own vault

7. Which of the following prescriptions are exempt from PPPA?

    A. Ambien (PA)
    B. Vibramycin (CR)

C. Ultram (ER)

D. Nitrostat (SL)

8. Which of the following medications are not indicated for the treatment of a patient with asthma?

A. Budesonide

B. Salbutamol

C. Ipratropium

D. Metoprolol

9. Spiriva, also known as an anticholinergic with the generic name of tiotropium, is used to treat which of the following conditions?

A. COPD

B. Hypertension

C. Diabetes

D. Congestive Heart Failure

10. You need to inject a STAT dose of 30 mg of Drug L. It is available as a 2.5% injectable solution. What is the volume that you will need to fulfill this prescription?

A. 0.6 ml

B. 9 ml

C. 12 ml

D. 1.2 ml

11. Which organization is dedicated to ensuring that errors are prevented, medication is used safely, and collects data from all the received reports from the Medication Errors Reporting Program (MERP)?

A. Academy of Managed Care Pharmacy (AMCP)

B. The Food and Drug Administration (FDA)

C. The Alliance for Safe Medication Awareness (ASMA)

D. Institute for Safe Medication Practices (ISMP)

12. A patient who needs Prevacid to be dispensed requests for a generic substitution. Which of the following drugs will you most likely dispense?

   A. Omeprazole
   B. Lansoprazole
   C. Sodium Citrate
   D. Ranitidine

13. Regarding a laminar flow clean bench, at which frequency should it be tested and accepted for proper airflow and particle collection?

   A. Every three months
   B. Every two weeks
   C. Annually
   D. Semi-annually

14. Which of the following drugs is considered to be a calcium channel blocker (CCB)?

   A. Carvedilol
   B. Simvastatin
   C. Verapamil
   D. Ranitidine

15. Child-resistant packaging is essential by law, per the PPPA. Which of the following drugs does not need to abide by this rule?

   A. Percocet 10/325
   B. Tylenol
   C. Ultram
   D. Loestrin

16. Medication that has been taken orally as its concentration is reduced due to its metabolism by the liver. What is this phenomenon whereby the drug is first metabolized by the GIT and liver systems?

   A. Redox Reaction

B. First Pass Effect

C. Zero Order Reaction

D. First Order Reaction

17. Which of the following drugs will need a new prescription and cannot be refilled?

A. Tylenol

B. Zolpidem

C. Methylphenidate

D. Ibuprofen

18. 18: Which of the following drugs is a DEA Schedule III?

A. Xanax

B. Lyrica

C. Tylenol

D. Androgel

19. Which of the following information regarding drugs can be referenced in the USP-National Formulary?

A. Storage requirements of drugs

B. The therapeutic equivalence of drugs

C. What the average wholesale price of a drug should be?

D. The scheduling of controlled substances

20. Which of the following temperatures is the nearest to the body temperature of humans?

A. 37 degrees Celsius

B. 41 degrees Celsius

C. 32 degrees Celsius

D. 25 degrees Celsius

21. Phentermine is known as a stimulant that acts by suppressing one's appetite. What schedule does phentermine fall under?

    A. Schedule I
    B. Schedule II
    C. Schedule IV
    D. Schedule III

22. For an OTC drug that costs $19.99 and is on special with a discount of 20% off, how much will it cost a patient who purchases two?

    A. $31.98
    B. $32.00
    C. $15.99
    D. $19.99

23. A patient with COPD is prescribed the Combivent Respimat. What is one of the active ingredients found in this inhaler?

    A. Tiotropium Bromide
    B. Aclidinium Bromide
    C. Ipratropium Bromide
    D. Uclidinium Bromide

24. Which of the following federal agencies will oversee the labeling, safety, and effectiveness of all products that can be placed in a compliant first aid kit?

    A. FDA
    B. OSHA
    C. DEA
    D. USP

25. You want to compound a patient's prescription but find the laminar flow hood has OObeen switched off. How long after switching it back on can you proceed with compounding?

    A. Immediately
    B. 15 minutes
    C. 30 minutes
    D. 45 minutes

26. A prescription requires a 2.25% solution of Drug A, but you only have 20 ml bottles of 6.75% strength in the pharmacy. If you place an entire bottle with distilled water, what will the final volume be?

    A. 70 ml
    B. 60 ml
    C. 50 ml
    D. 40 ml

27. What is the name of the dosage form where the tablet slowly disintegrates in a patient's mouth?

    A. Douche
    B. Troche
    C. Sucreter
    D. Droppie

28. You need to give the patient a 2.75% syrup, and they weigh 121 lbs. It is ordered to be taken at 5 mg/kg Q12H #10. If the solution comes in 6 fl oz bottles, how many would you need to dispense?

    A. One
    B. Two
    C. Three
    D. Four

29. Which of the following side effects is common with an ACE Inhibitor?

    A. Dry cough
    B. Hair loss
    C. A buildup of ear wax
    D. Irritability

30. For how many years must you keep records of all prescriptions containing controlled substances?

    A. 2 Years
    B. 3 Years
    C. 4 Years
    D. 5 Years

31. You spill a chemical, and it starts to emit a noxious odor. What is the first thing you should do to comply with the spill-handling procedure?

    A. Clean it up without gloves
    B. Pull the fire alarm
    C. Throw water over it
    D. Consult the drug's MSDS document

32. You receive a prescription for Vicodin 1 tab QID PRN #7. How many refills can the script be written for if the prescriber has legally requested repeats?

    A. Six refills and today's filling
    B. Two refills within 90 days of the script date
    C. No refills
    D. Five refills within 6 months of the script's date

33. Which of the following concentrations of NaCl is isotonic?

    A. 0.9%
    B. 9%
    C. 0.09%

D. 0.009%

34. You are requested to create "Compound Q," which needs to be divided into 0.25 Kg parts. Its recipe is as follows: S is 7.5 parts, K is 8.0 parts, D is 9.0 parts, and O is 25.5 parts. How much of ingredient K will be needed for the batch?

    A. 70 grams
    B. 64 grams
    C. 50 grams
    D. 40 grams

35. What do you call a bacterial infection that was obtained in the hospital?

    A. Community-acquired infection
    B. Nosocomial infection
    C. Sanitorial infection
    D. Pharyngeal infection

36. How much pseudoephedrine can a patient purchase in a 30-day period from a single pharmacy in accordance with the CMEA Act of 2005?

    A. 7 grams
    B. 8 grams
    C. 9 grams
    D. 9.5 grams

37. Unopened insulin needs to be stored in a refrigerator. What is the correct temperature it should be stored at?

    A. 0 to 14 degrees Fahrenheit
    B. 36 to 46 degrees Fahrenheit
    C. 34 to 43 degrees Celsius
    D. 28 to 32 degrees Fahrenheit

38. Which of the following is not a benefit when we compare tablets with other dosage forms?

    A. Rapid onset of action
    B. A longer shelf life
    C. Much easier to administer
    D. Has a more accurate form of dosing

39. In terms of pharmacokinetics, what is the pathway a drug will take?

    A. Distribution, Elimination, Absorption, Metabolism
    B. Metabolism, Distribution, Absorption, Elimination
    C. Absorption, Metabolism, Distribution, Elimination
    D. Absorption, Distribution, Metabolism, Elimination

40. Amoxicillin present in 250 mg/5 ml is given to a child prescribed a dose of 100 mg BD PO. How many ml should be administered per dose?

    A. 2 ml
    B. 2.5 ml
    C. 3 ml
    D. 3.5 ml

41. What does it mean when a drug is prescribed for "off-label" use?

    A. It is not used for its intended purpose as per FDA-approved indications for that drug.
    B. The term does not exist.
    C. The generic drug is to be prescribed but at a higher cost than the brand name.
    D. You are allowed to change the dosage form without asking for the patient's permission.

42. You see a patient who brings you a script for ofloxacin 0.3%/10 ml. It reads: 5 gtt AD BID X10D. What will you write on the label?

    A. Instill 5 drops into both ears twice per day for 10 days.

B. Instill 5 drops into both eyes twice per day for 10 days.

C. Instill 5 drops into the right ear twice daily for 10 days.

D. Instill 5 drops into the left ear twice daily for 10 days.

43. Which of the following drugs is allowed to not be placed in a child-proof container?

   A. Metformin
   B. Nitroglycerin
   C. Sildenafil
   D. Amoxicillin

44. Which of the following drugs are contraindicated in patients who are currently using warfarin?

   A. Prednisone
   B. Aspirin
   C. Enalapril
   D. Amlodipine

45. Which of the following does not need to be included on unit-dose package labels?

   A. NDC Number
   B. Expiry date
   C. Lot number
   D. Strength of the medication

46. How many days should the following lithium prescription last? It reads: Lithium 300 mg #90, 1 tab Q8H PO.

   A. 15 days
   B. 45 days
   C. 30 days
   D. 60 days

47. Which of the following DEA forms need to be completed if there is loss or theft of a controlled substance?

    A. DEA Form 101
    B. DEA Form 102
    C. DEA Form 105
    D. DEA Form 106

48. Drug T has an annual inventory turnover rate of 9.2 which is higher than the previous year. What is this number?

    A. The number of times Drug T was sold and replaced throughout the year.
    B. The number of boxes of Drug T expired throughout the year.
    C. How many employees who dealt with Drug T were terminated throughout the year?
    D. The price of Drug T per order throughout the year.

49. What is the recommended dosage, as stipulated by the FDA, that acetaminophen should not exceed?

    A. 1 gram over a 24-hour period
    B. 2 grams over a 24-hour period
    C. 3 grams over a 24-hour period
    D. 4 grams over a 24-hour period

50. Which of the following is known as "birth control?"

    A. Loestrin
    B. Seroquel
    C. Xanax
    D. Evista

51. What is the name of drugs that are present on a list based on their economic and therapeutic considerations?

    A. The orange list
    B. The FDA-approved drug list

C. A formulary

D. An economic-therapeutic list

52. What is the name of the authoritative body that is responsible for ensuring that USP<797> standards and violations are enforced?

A. BOP

B. JCAHO

C. FDA

D. USP

53. Which of the following is an absolute requirement for any drug order before it is dispensed to the patient?

A. It should contain a patient package insert.

B. It should be in a child-proof container.

C. The patient should have a negative pregnancy test.

D. Pharmacist-conducted counseling has been performed.

54. What drug class is Vasotec a part of?

A. Diuretics

B. Antibiotics

C. ACE Inhibitors

D. Benzodiazepines

55. Which term is used to describe the process that a drug's rate of absorption occurs, delivering the drug to the proper site in the body to perform its action?

A. Efficacy

B. Potency

C. Inhibition

D. Bioavailability

56. A script for Drug L is given to you, and it reads: 20 mg BD PO x14D. You only have 10 mg tablets in stock. How many would you count to fulfill this prescription order?

    A. 28 tablets
    B. 72 tablets
    C. 56 tablets
    D. 112 tablets

57. A 1L Viaflex container of 20 mEq/L KCl in D5NS has the following NDC number: 0338-0803-04. Approximately how much NaCl is within this product?

    A. 900 mcg
    B. 900 mg
    C. 9000 mg
    D. 8 ounces

58. Which of the following elements is not classified as being an electrolyte?

    A. Dextrose
    B. Magnesium sulfate
    C. Potassium chloride
    D. Sodium chloride

59. What is the brand name for verapamil?

    A. Coreg
    B. Norvasc
    C. Calan
    D. Cardizem

60. How does the following sig code string read: 1 tsp QID PO PC et HS?

    A. One teaspoon by mouth every 6 hours, both before meals and at bedtime
    B. One teaspoon by mouth every 6 hours, both after meals and at bedtime
    C. One teaspoon by mouth every 2 hours, both before meals and at bedtime

D. Two teaspoons by mouth every 4 hours, both after meals and at bedtime

61. What do the last two digits present in the NDC number indicate?

   A. Manufacturer
   B. Expiration date
   C. Lot number
   D. Package size

62. You are using a pipette dropper in a graduated cylinder. After approximately 31 drops, you have reached the 2.5 ml mark. How many ml are there in each drop?

   A. 0.1 ml
   B. 0.09 ml
   C. 0.08 ml
   D. 0.07 ml

63. Given a prescription for latanoprost (0.005% solution) that reads: 1 gtt OU QPM, what auxiliary label would you ensure goes on the packaging?

   A. For the eyes
   B. For the skin
   C. Take one tablet until the course is complete
   D. Put one drop in both ears twice per day

64. A six-year-old patient who weighs 44 lbs needs a drug dosed at 15 mg/Kg/Day and needs to receive BD. How much drug will the child receive with each dose?

   A. 150 mg
   B. 300 mg
   C. 75 mg
   D. 600 mg

65. Which of the following drugs is considered a beta-2 agonist?

    A. Tiotropium
    B. Carvedilol
    C. Enalapril
    D. Albuterol

66. What is the brand name for simvastatin?

    A. Simvachol
    B. Pravachol
    C. Zocor
    D. Lipocor

67. Which of the following agencies outlines all MSDS disclosure requirements?

    A. DEA
    B. FDA
    C. PTCB
    D. OSHA

68. A PTCB qualification needs to be renewed every two years. Which of the following does not meet the continuing education needs for CPhT recertification?

    A. One hour of patient safety
    B. One hour of aseptic technique training
    C. One hour of law
    D. Twenty hours of clinical work

69. Which drug would you prescribe to treat hypercholesterolemia?

    A. Tricor
    B. Lotrisone
    C. Ultram
    D. Zyprexa

70. What condition would one typically use nystatin for?

    A. Oral candidiasis
    B. Nasal infection
    C. Ear infection
    D. Throat infection

71. If a patient is covered by more than one health insurance plan, what method is implemented to see which of the insurance plans will pay the main amount and which will pay the remaining costs?

    A. Sequential Plan Billing (SPB)
    B. Coordination of Benefits (COB)
    C. Claim Ratio Adjustment (CRA)
    D. Food and Drug Administration Allocation (FDAA)

72. Which of the following drugs can be used to lower both your triglyceride and cholesterol levels?

    A. Vytorin
    B. Ultram
    C. Cardizem
    D. Tarigen

73. A prescription you receive wants 120 ml of a 0.5% solution. You have 100 x 50 mg tablets in a count bottle. How many tablets will you need to fulfill this prescription?

    A. 3 tablets
    B. 6 tablets
    C. 9 tablets
    D. 12 tablets

74. Which of the following auxiliary labels will you ensure is on all prescriptions that contain a tetracycline?

    A. Do not expose to sunlight

B. Do not take it with dairy

C. Make sure to take it with food

D. Make sure to take it on an empty stomach

75. The wholesale cost of a bulk container of 1,000 tablets of Drug X is $100. What would the retail price of 90 tablets be given the pharmacy uses a 25% markup and adds a $3.25 dispensing fee?

A. $115.75

B. $144.65

C. $142.51

D. $153.67

76. Which of the following is not an anti-diabetic drug?

A. Byetta

B. Actos

C. Januvia

D. Lyrica

77. Which of the following is present in the Orange Book?

A. The average price of all drugs when purchased from different wholesalers

B. The generic equivalents for all the brand-name drugs

C. The dosage recommendation

D. All drug-drug interactions

78. An elderly patient comes to you and says after taking a specific OTC drug, she started feeling sharp chest pains. What would you advise her to do?

A. Go to an emergency room immediately

B. Take your time and consult the pharmacist

C. Call 911 and give her some aspirin

D. Inject her with an EpiPen

79. Which of the following orders can be compounded safely using the aseptic technique?

    A. Etoposide injection
    B. Hydrocodone/APAP tablet counting
    C. Ampicillin suspension
    D. Mupirocin cream

80. The generic name for Plavix is clopidogrel. What class does it fall under?

    A. Platelet aggregate inhibitor
    B. Antidepressant
    C. Antidiabetic
    D. Antihyperlipidemic

81. Which of the following drugs is not a diuretic?

    A. Furosemide
    B. Spironolactone
    C. Hydrochlorothiazide
    D. Lamotrigine

82. Which of the following drugs is used as estrogen replacement therapy?

    A. Restoril
    B. Ultram
    C. Premarin
    D. Lioresal

83. Ibuprofen is known as an:

    A. Antihypertensive
    B. Antidiabetic
    C. NSAID
    D. DMARD

84. With regards to federal law, for how long should all DEA form 222s be held in the pharmacy?

   A. 2 years
   B. 3 years
   C. 4 years
   D. 7 years

85. What is the role of hydrochlorothiazide?

   A. To prevent urinary tract infections
   B. To increase serotonin levels in your brain
   C. To inhibit the body's ability to retain water, preventing loading on the cardiac system
   D. Treats erectile dysfunction

86. Regarding Clark's rule, what is a factor that is used to calculate a child's dose from an adult's dose?

   A. Body surface area
   B. Adult's age
   C. Weight in pounds
   D. Weight in kilograms

87. Isotretinoin can cause immense complications in pregnancy. What is the name of the program which prevents women who are or want to become pregnant from being exposed to the drug?

   A. AWARxE
   B. SMART
   C. SAFEPreg
   D. iPLEDGE

88. Which of the following needles is less likely to cause coring of a vial's rubber stopper?

   A. 20 gauge

B. 18 gauge

C. 16 gauge

D. 12 gauge

89. What DEA Schedule are Adderall and Vyvanse?

A. Schedule II

B. Schedule III

C. Schedule IV

D. Schedule V

90. What number do the roman numerals XIV refer to?

A. 104

B. 14

C. 4

D. 140

Answer Key

Q.	1	2	3	4	5	6	7	8	9	10
A.	A	B	B	C	B	B	D	D	A	D

Q.	11	12	13	14	15	16	17	18	19	20
A.	D	B	D	C	D	B	C	D	A	A

Q.	21	22	23	24	25	26	27	28	29	30
A.	C	A	C	A	C	B	B	B	A	A

Q.	31	32	33	34	35	36	37	38	39	40
A.	D	C	A	D	B	C	B	A	D	A

Q.	41	42	43	44	45	46	47	48	49	50
A.	A	C	B	B	A	C	D	A	D	A

Q.	51	52	53	54	55	56	57	58	59	60
A.	C	A	A	C	D	A	C	A	C	B

Q.	61	62	63	64	65	66	67	68	69	70
A.	D	C	A	A	D	C	D	B	A	A

Q.	71	72	73	74	75	76	77	78	79	80
A.	B	A	D	C	A	D	B	A	A	A

Q.	81	82	83	84	85	86	87	88	89	90
A.	D	C	C	A	C	C	D	A	A	B

Answer Explanations

1.   A: A liquid is best for those with swallowing difficulties.

2.   B: Ophthalmic preparations are usually in an ointment or drop dosage form.

3.   B: Stock rotation ensures the products closest to expiry are used first.

4.   C: To calculate this effectively, you need to be able to convert cc to ml. You will then be able to see how many total hours 25,000 units of heparin will run over using the converted amount of the total solution.

5.   B: Ultram's generic name is tramadol hydrochloride.

6.   B: A refrigerator will give the required temperature. Not in the freezer!

7.   D: Nitrostat is needed in some emergencies, and so does not need to follow PPPA regulations.

8.   D: Metoprolol is a beta blocker and is contraindicated in patients with asthma.

9.   A: Tiotropium is used to treat COPD.

10.   D: Expressing the 2.5% as a percentage strength will allow you to compare ingredient amounts with each other and solve for "x" to get the answer.

11.   D: ISMP ensures drugs are used safely and aims to prevent errors through received reports from MERP.

12.   B: Lansoprazole is the generic name for Prevacid.

13.   D: A laminar flow clean bench should be tested semi-annually.

14.   C: Verapamil is an example of a calcium channel blocker.

15.   D: Loestrin is an oral contraceptive and is exempt from the PPPA rules.

16. B: The first metabolism of a drug by the liver and GIT system is known as the First Pass Effect or First Pass Metabolism.

17. C: Methylphenidate is DEA Schedule II and will always need a new prescription for it to be dispensed. It cannot be refilled, and no repeats can be allocated.

18. D: Androgel is an example of a DEA Schedule III drug.

19. A: The storage requirements of drugs can be found in the USP-NE.

20. A: 37 degrees Celsius is the closest to the human body temperature of 36.5 to 37.5 degrees Celsius.

21. C: Phentermine is considered a DEA Schedule IV drug.

22. A: Here, the best way to approach it is to calculate 20% of the $19.99 and then multiply it by two.

23. C: Ipratropium Bromide is found in Combivent Respimat.

24. A: The FDA is responsible for overseeing the labeling, safety, and effectiveness of all first aid products.

25. C: You need to wait 30 minutes after switching on a laminar flow hood before you can start compounding.

26. B: By equating the two percentage strengths together, you can solve for "x" to obtain the final volume.

27. B: A troche is the name of a dosage form that slowly disintegrates in the mouth.

28. B: Here, it is recommended to convert your fl oz to ml, as well as your lbs to Kg. This way, you can calculate the answer using constant units of measurement.

29. A: A common side effect of ACE inhibitors is a dry cough.

30. A: All prescription records need to be kept for at least two years.

31. D: Consulting the drug's MSDS document will tell you exactly what to do regarding that specific drug.

32. C: Vicodin is a drug that cannot qualify for refills.

33. A: Isotonic means "neutral," which would be the concentration that NaCl usually comes in. This is 0.9%.

34. D: Total up the number of parts, divide K's parts by the total amount, and multiply it by 250 grams to get the answer.

35. B: Nosocomial infections are those picked up in the hospital during the period a patient is admitted.

36. C: A total of 9 grams of pseudoephedrine can be purchased over a 30-day period as per the CMEA Act of 2005.

37. B: Unopened insulin needs to be present in the refrigerator, which is between 2 and 14 degrees Celsius.

38. A: Tablets do not provide a rapid onset of action.

39. D: The acronym ADME stands for Absorption, Distribution, Metabolism, Excretion.

40. A: Simplify the 250 mg/5 ml to 1 ml and then multiply that amount of active ingredient by a factor to get 100 mg. The answer will be the dose amount that needs to be administered.

41. A: Off-label use is using a drug for a reason other than its approved FDA indication.

42. C: The key here is to know that AD means the right ear.

43. B: Nitroglycerin is used in emergencies and does not need to be placed in a child-proof container.

44. B: Aspirin is contraindicated in patients using warfarin as it prevents platelets from clotting wounds.

45. A: The NDC number does not need to be on unit-dose package labels.

46. C: Being able to read that the dosing is ever 8 hours and that 90 tablets are to be given will allow you to calculate the answer as a 30-day supply.

47. 47 - D: The DEA Form 106 needs to be completed in the cases of the theft or loss of controlled substances.

48. A: The annual inventory turnover ratio tells you how many of a specific product was sold and then replaced during the year.

49. D: Acetaminophen's dose is 1 gram every 6 hours, totaling a maximum of 4 grams per day.

50. A: Loestrin is known as an oral contraceptive or "birth control."

51. C: A formulary is a list of drugs based on their therapeutic and economic viability.

52. A: The State Board of Pharmacists (BOP) ensures USP <797> standards and violations are enforced.

53. A: A package insert should always accompany a patient when dispensing medication.

54. C: Vasotec is an ACE inhibitor.

55. D: Bioavailability will tell you what percentage of drug taken is available for use by the body after the first pass effect has taken place.

56. A: You have half the required dose in stock, so you take the total for the script and multiply it by two to get the answer.

57. C: Here, you need to know your conversions, especially the mEq conversions.

58. A: Dextrose is not an electrolyte.

59. C: Verapamil's brand name is Calan.

60. B: The trick here is knowing that PC means after meals and that HS means at bedtime.

61. D: The last two digits of the NDC number tell you the package size.

62. C: 1 ml = approximately 20 drops. This is the important conversion you need to know to get to the answer.

63. A: For the eyes will be on the auxiliary label.

64. A: Here, you will need to convert lbs to Kg to solve this equation.

65. D: Albuterol is a beta-2 agonist.

66. C: Simvastatin's brand name is Zocor.

67. D: All MSDS disclosure requirements are outlined in OSHA.

68. B: An hour of aseptic technique training does not fulfill the continuing education requirements for renewing your PTCB qualification.

69. A: Tricor is used to treat hypercholesterolemia.

70. A: Nystatin is typically used to treat oral candidiasis.

71. B: Coordination of Benefits (COB) will decide which insurance plan pays the main amount and which pays for the shortfall (if any).

72. A: Vytorin will assist in lowering both your triglyceride and cholesterol levels.

73. D: Calculating the mg by expanding the 0.5% into its constituents will enable you to calculate the total of 12 tablets needed to achieve the required

volume of the concentration.

74. C: Tetracyclines need to be taken with food.

75. A: By calculating the wholesale price of 90 tablets, you can easily calculate the percentage markup and add the dispensing fee.

76. D: Lyrica is not an antidiabetic drug.

77. B: The generic equivalents of all drugs are present in the Orange Book.

78. A: The reaction could be lethal, so the recommendation is always to go to the emergency room. You want to err on the side of caution!

79. A: Etopside injections can be compounded safely aseptically.

80. A: Clopidogrel is a platelet aggregate inhibitor.

81. D: Lamotrigine is not a diuretic.

82. C: Premarin is used as estrogen replacement therapy.

83. C: Ibuprofen is a NSAID.

84. A: All DEA Form 222s need to be kept for at least 2 years.

85. C: Hydrochlorothiazide is a diuretic, meaning it makes sure fluid is not retained in the body.

86. C: Clark's rule requires the weights of both the adults and child in lbs.

87. D: iPLEDGE is the name of the isotretinoin program.

88. A: The greater the gauge number, the smaller the diameter.

89. A: Adderall and Vyvanse are DEA Schedule II.

90. B: XIV is 14.

Chapter Seven: Full-Length Practice Test #2

Questions

1. Which one of the FDA-approved recalls is one where the patient may experience temporary adverse effects due to the medication?

   A. Class I
   B. Class II
   C. Class III
   D. Class IV

2. Which of these is seen as being acceptable storage means for prescription records?

   A. Two different files. One for Controlled Schedule II and one for Non-Controlled Schedule III to V.
   B. Three files. One for Controlled Schedule II to III and a Non-Controlled file.
   C. Two files. One for Controlled Schedule II and Non-Controled, and another for Controlled Schedule III to V.
   D. One file. Contains everything.

3. What is the appropriate form that can be used to order your controlled substances from a supplier?

    A. DEA form 222
    B. DEA form 224
    C. DEA form 106
    D. DEA form 101

4. Which of the following DEA numbers are valid?

    A. CG2467896
    B. CG2467895
    C. CG2467894
    D. CG2467892

5. How many years will a prescription need to be retained onsite by a particular state's pharmacy?

    A. Depending on the state, two to five years
    B. Ten years across all of the states
    C. Depending on the state, five to eight years
    D. Depending on the state, one to three years

6. Which of the following statements can always be considered true regarding your Schedule II controlled substances?

    A. They must always be ordered using a DEA form 222 that is handwritten.
    B. The pharmacist who is in charge needs to always document and verify the date of all received Schedule II controlled medications.
    C. The destruction of Schedule II drugs can only be done if a DEA agent is present.
    D. Once received by the pharmacy, a Schedule II drug cannot be returned to the supplier for reverse distribution.

7. When receiving transferred Schedule III to V medications, what needs to be documented by the pharmacy receiving the medication?

    A. The date on which the prescription expires
    B. The transferring pharmacy's DEA number
    C. The format of the original prescription
    D. The date of birth of the patient

8. If a patient purchases pseudoephedrine, what needs to be placed into the logbook?

    A. The total amount purchased
    B. The day of the week that it was purchased
    C. The date of birth of the purchaser
    D. The last date that the purchaser purchased more pseudoephedrine

9. What set of standards ensures all pharmacy employees are kept safe while doing their duties?

    A. USP 795
    B. OSHA
    C. HIPAA
    D. PPA

10. Regarding the disposal of hazardous drug waste, which of the following is true?

    A. Disposal must occur within 48 hours.
    B. All drug waste must be stored together until properly disposed of.
    C. It must be put in a leakproof container.
    D. Its label must read "drug waste."

11. If the federal pharmacy law and the state's pharmacy law conflict with each other, which law should be followed?

    A. The law which is more strict
    B. The law which is less strict

C. The state's law

D. The federal pharmacy law

12. All of the following statements are common reasons for recalling medication except for:

A. Mislabeling of products

B. Impurity presence

C. Cost of medication.

D. Contamination of medication

13. What is the acronym that depicts the online platform for ordering controlled substances?

A. AMPA

B. PMP

C. CSOS

D. REMS

14. The CMEA Act of 2005 restricts all of the following medications except—

A. Pseudoephedrine

B. Ephedrine

C. Phenylephrine

D. Phenylpropanolamine

15. Toprol is the brand name for—

A. Atenolol

B. Carvedilol

C. Metoprolol

D. Propranolol

16. You receive a prescription for Paxil 10mg QD. Which medication and dosing are being asked for?

A. Paroxetine 10mg once daily.

B. Fluoxetine 10mg once daily.

C. Escitalopram 10mg once daily

D. Citalopram 10mg once daily.

17. How should patients take a sublingual tablet?

A. Place it against their cheeks.

B. Swallow it whole.

C. Place it under their tongue.

D. Chew the tablet and swallow it.

18. Which of the following instructions is in keeping with the administration of enteral medication?

A. Inhale

B. Inject

C. Apply

D. Swallow

19. Which of the following dosage forms need to be shaken well before administration?

A. Insulin vial.

B. An injectablet.

C. Otic suspension.

D. Oral solution.

20. What is Zoloft's generic name?

A. Amlodipine

B. Sitagliptin

C. Simethicone

D. Sertraline

21. A patient has just undergone surgery and is taking both Percocet and Tylenol. Which of the following active ingredients is present in both of these medications?

    A. Hydrocodone
    B. Acetaminophen
    C. Ibuprofen
    D. Oxycodone

22. The FDA advises females of child-bearing age to not use Finasteride as it has a high potential of harming the fetus. What type of warning is this an example of?

    A. Adverse event
    B. Allergy
    C. Drug-supplement interaction
    D. Contraindication

23. Which route of administration should a suppository follow?

    A. Topical
    B. Intramuscular
    C. Rectal
    D. Oral

24. A patient takes a drug and experiences muscle weakness shortly afterward. What medication-related problem is the patient experiencing?

    A. Side effect
    B. Allergy
    C. A therapeutic contraindication
    D. A drug-drug interaction

25. What is a common side effect that is experienced by patients who take diphenhydramine?

    A. Neuropathic pain

B. Drowsiness

C. Liver failure

D. Diarrhea

26. Overdose of which drug can cause liver failure?

    A. Aspirin
    B. Ibuprofen
    C. Naproxen
    D. Acetaminophen

27. Which of the following pain relievers contains acetaminophen?

    A. Roxicet
    B. Roxicodone
    C. Percodan
    D. Oxycontin

28. How many days is a water-based oral solution stable for?

    A. 7 days
    B. 10 days
    C. 14 days
    D. 21 days

29. Which of the following is not seen as being a sign of incompatibility?

    A. Precipitate formation
    B. Color change
    C. Unexpected cloudiness
    D. Nonuniform product

30. If gentamicin comes in 80 mg/2 ml vials, how many will be needed for an IV bag that needs to contain 480 mg of gentamicin

    A. 3 vials
    B. 6 vials

C. 9 vials

D. 12 vials

31. If the infusion rate is 3–5 hours for a 500 ml bag, what is the rate of infusion?

    A. 30.3 ml/min

    B. 3.3 ml/min

    C. 2.38 ml/min

    D. 23.8 ml/min

32. If octreotide is only available in vials of 1,000 mcg/5 mls, how many mls are needed for an IV bag to contain 600 mcg?

    A. 1 ml

    B. 2 ml

    C. 3 ml

    D. 4 ml

33. If your plan as a pharmacy technician is to run medication over 12 hours, how many milliliters do you need if the infusion runs at 1 ml per minute?

    A. 720 ml

    B. 7,200 ml

    C. 500 ml

    D. 5,000 ml

34. In which cases should an expiration date be present?

    A. All drugs

    B. Only OTC

    C. Only prescription

    D. Only liquids

35. What is the therapeutic substitution of a drug?

   A. Substitution of a drug with one from a different class but that will provide the same effects.
   B. Substitution of a drug for another drug because the initial one is too expensive.
   C. Substitution of a drug with another drug because it is not as popular as the initial drug.
   D. Substitution of a drug for another drug because the brand name and generic names are not available.

36. If a prescriber states "dispense as written," how should you dispense it?

   A. Use only the brand names
   B. Use only generic names
   C. Ask the patient what they want
   D. Ask the pharmacist what is best

37. If no specific storage requirements are on a drug, what temperature should it be kept at?

   A. 10 to 20 degrees Fahrenheit
   B. 25 to 45 degrees Fahrenheit
   C. 55 to 66 degrees Fahrenheit
   D. 68 to 77 degrees Fahrenheit

38. Once a drug is approved, who will monitor the drug's safety?

   A. The patient
   B. The pharmacist
   C. The manufacturer
   D. The FDA

39. Of the following drugs, which one has a narrow therapeutic index?

   A. Acetaminophen
   B. Lisinopril

C. Pantoprazole

D. Warfarin

40. Which of the following can be referred to as a true allergy?

A. Diarrhea

B. Constipation

C. Hives

D. Altered cognition

41. Regarding insulin, what is its standard concentration?

A. 100 units/ml

B. 200 units/ml

C. 300 units/ml

D. 400 units/ml

42. Which drug class has the suffix -pyrazole?

A. Angiotensin blockers

B. Beta blockers

C. PPIs

D. ACE inhibitors

43. One tablespoon of liquid is equal to how many mls?

A. 10 ml

B. 15 ml

C. 20 ml

D. 25 ml

44. Given the following prescription: 1 gtt OU QPM, how many days would 2.5 ml of an eye drop container last?

A. 25 days

B. 30 days

C. 20 days

D. 18 days

45.   400 mcg of folic acid is equal to how many mg?

A. 40 mg
B. 4 mg
C. 0.4 mg
D. 0.04 mg

46.   You are required to make 420 ml of a 25% solution. How many mls of a 40% and 12% solution will you need?

A. 298 ml of a 40% solution and 122 ml of a 12% solution
B. 195 ml of a 40% solution and 225 ml of a 12% solution
C. 90 ml of a 40% solution and 330 ml of a 12% solution
D. 245 ml of a 40% solution and 175 ml of a 12% solution

47.   Regarding all compounded products, what always needs to be documented?

A. The NDC number
B. The initials of the pharmacy manager
C. Whether the compound has come from a batch that has been premixed.
D. Lot number.

48.   When compounding a single prescription, how many people should be involved?

A. One
B. Two
C. Three
D. Four

49.   What would the w/w% be of 412.5 mg of nitroglycerin that is placed in 33 grams of a compounded prescription?

A. 0.0125% nitroglycerin
B. 0.125% nitroglycerin

    C. 1.25% nitroglycerin

    D. 12.5% nitroglycerin

50.   You are required to make 800 ml of a 25% solution. How many mls of a 30% and 10% solution will you need?

    A. 600 ml of a 30% solution and 200 ml of a 10% solution

    B. 490 ml of a 30% solution and 310 ml of a 10% solution

    C. 560 ml of a 30% solution and 240 ml of a 10% solution

    D. 650 ml of a 30% solution and 150 ml of a 10% solution

51.   When you are performing non-sterile compounding, when should you put on your PPE?

    A. After collecting and organizing all of your hardware

    B. After you have received the prescription

    C. After you have weighed and measured all of the ingredients

    D. After you have done all of the calculations and formulas

52.   What is the w/v% of 0.5 grams of Drug D in 50 ml of a solution?

    A. 1% w/v

    B. 2% w/v

    C. 5% w/v

    D. 10% w/v

53.   Regarding legal requirements, which specific piece of compounding equipment must be present in each and every pharmacy?

    A. Laminar flow hood

    B. Class A prescription balance

    C. Syringes

    D. Three different types of mortar and pestle

54. When processing a prescription, there are five steps to it. However, which of them can only be performed by a pharmacist?

A. Translation of the prescription
B. Verifying the prescription during the patient consultation
C. Filling the prescription
D. Receiving the prescription

55. You receive a script for Cipro 500 mg 1 Tab PO BID for 10 days. How many tablets would you need to dispense with fulfilling the prescription?

A. 20 tablets
B. 24 tablets
C. 30 tablets
D. 36 tablets

56. Translate the following prescription: 1 Cap PO AC TID:

A. One capsule by mouth before meals three times a day
B. Once capsule by mouth after meals three times a day
C. One capsule by mouth three times a day
D. One capsule by mouth before and after meals three times a day

57. As a pharmacy technician, which of the following is not in your scope of practice?

A. Ensuring the accuracy of a drug by looking at its NDC number
B. Reconstituting a drug before the pharmacist signs off on it
C. Counting out drugs and placing them in a bottle
D. Labeling of a prescription bottle

58. What is the NDC number?

A. An 11-digit number
B. A 12-digit number
C. An 8-digit number
D. A 9-digit number

59. Assuming that Humalog U-100 comes in 10 ml vials, how many days of supply will you have if the patient injects 10 U SQ QID?

    A. 20 days
    B. 25 days
    C. 50 days
    D. 100 days

60. Translate the following: 1 gtt OS BID:

    A. Instill one drop into both ears twice daily
    B. Instill two drops into the left eye once daily
    C. Instill one drop into the left eye twice daily
    D. Instill one drop into both eyes twice daily

61. What is a lot number?

    A. A 10-digit number that will tell you information about the manufacturer
    B. What is used to identify a drug's package size?
    C. What drug is given through the manufacturing process in case of a recall.
    D. A number that tells you the dosage form of a drug

62. In which of the following instances does a drug not need to be quarantined?

    A. The drug bottle is open
    B. The drug comes from a rather questionable source
    C. The drug has been recalled
    D. The patient has returned the prescription

63. What is the term for the following: "Any preventable event that may cause or lead to inappropriate medication use or patient harm while the medication is in the control of the healthcare professional, patient, or consumer?"

    A. Knowledge deficit
    B. Performance deficit
    C. Prescription abuse
    D. Medication error

64.   Which process is recommended to avoid transcription errors?

    A. All high-risk drugs need to have associated indications
    B. All phone orders must be repeated before ending the call
    C. A zero should always be included after a decimal point
    D. Require a double-check of an independent dose

65.   Which of the following situations is an example of the unintentional misuse of medication?

    A. The patient continues to take opioids even though they no longer need them.
    B. A patient takes benzodiazepines three times per day instead of just before flying.
    C. The patient makes use of their rescue inhaler multiple times per day instead of just when emergency shortness of breath occurs.
    D. A patient uses another person's prescription to self-medicate.

66.   Which of the following organizations has authority over all of the high-alert medications that are present across the different healthcare settings?

    A. The Institute for Safe Medication Practices
    B. DEA
    C. FDA
    D. Substance Abuse and Mental Health Administration Center for Behavioral Health Statistics and Quality

67.   What is the term that we use to describe a drug that has the potential to cause considerable harm when it is used in error?

    A. Prescription abuse
    B. Drug-drug interactions
    C. High-alert medications
    D. Adverse drug events

68. Tall man lettering is the most appropriate for which pair of drugs?

    A. Digoxin/Lopinavir
    B. Ritonavir/Repaglinide
    C. Metoclopramide/Omeprazole
    D. Hydralazine/Hydroxyzine

69. Which of the below-mentioned scenarios can attribute to a prescriber error?

    A. Illegible handwriting
    B. Using floor stock instead of medications in single-unit doses
    C. Borrowing medication from a different patient
    D. Bypassing the use of a barcoded administration system

70. Which of the following medication orders would be seen as the most appropriate to be used?

    A. Take one tab QD
    B. Tk 1 tab PO QD
    C. 1 tab per os QD
    D. Take one tablet by mouth daily

71. Which of the following is an example of a trailing zero?

    A. 5.1
    B. 5.0
    C. 500
    D. 0.05

72. Which of the following medication orders would be seen as the most appropriate to be used?

    A. Take 10 mg of medicine per os twice daily
    B. 10 mg twice daily
    C. Take 10 mg by mouth twice daily
    D. Take 10.0 mg PO BD

73. Which of the following notions is present on the Institute for Safe Medication Practice's list for dose designation, symbols, and abbreviations?

    A. PO
    B. HS
    C. un
    D. Once daily

74. Which of the following notions is present on the Institute for Safe Medication Practice's list for dose designation, symbols, and abbreviations?

    A. cc
    B. L
    C. units
    D. mcg

75. If a patient is admitted to the hospital on Drug Y and is switched to Drug X, what would this be seen as?

    A. Misuse
    B. Equivalence
    C. Therapeutic interchange
    D. OTC recommendation

76. You see a prescription that says the following: "Take one Zoloft tablet by mouth daily." What is missing?

    A. The strength of the drug
    B. The route
    C. The drug name
    D. The frequency

77. What is it called when a caregiver forgets to give their patient their medication?

    A. Intentional misuse
    B. Missed dose

C. Therapeutic interchange

D. Adverse drug event

78. Regarding Continuous Quality Improvement (CQI), what is its primary purpose?

A. To speed up the workflow

B. To ensure healthcare accreditation standards are met

C. To improve all pharmacy practices

D. To create punitive judgment over employee medication errors

79. When a medication error occurs, what is the first step to complete?

A. Treat the patient should they have any side effects

B. Document the error

C. Utilise quality assurance practices to see what went wrong

D. Report the error to the district manager

80. Of the following organizations, which one lists all the inappropriate abbreviations that assist pharmacy personnel against making medication errors?

A. FDA

B. OSHA

C. DEA

D. ISMP

81. When looking at quality assurance when compounding, what is the most important aspect of PPE?

A. Appropriate handwashing technique and frequency

B. Taking off all jewelry after PPE is donned

C. Starting with the facemask

D. Recapping all needles

82. What benefit does the barcode system supply the pharmacy with?

    A. Assist in establishing good inventory values
    B. Improves workflow efficiency
    C. Verification of drug products before reaching the patient
    D. Optimize everything relating to data entry processes

83. Which of the following will not act toward improving the safety of medication?

    A. Punishing all staff members who make medication errors
    B. Ensuring adequate personal health and hygiene
    C. Standardizing all pharmacy workflow
    D. Automation and computerization of processes

84. Regarding PPE, which of the following is appropriate?

    A. When donning PPE, work dirtiest to cleanest
    B. Wearing a watch is fine if it fits in your glove
    C. Gloves are always the first item donned
    D. Always put your facemask on first

85. Which of the following pharmacy staff members can ask the patient if they would like counseling from a pharmacist regarding their medication?

    A. Pharmacist
    B. Pharmacy technician
    C. Pharmacy intern
    D. All of the above

86. Which of the following is a task that can only be performed by a pharmacist?

    A. Entering new prescriptions onto the computerized database
    B. Maintaining all of the medication inventory
    C. Ensuring that there is transfer of a prescription via an unshared network
    D. Compounding products

87. Regarding the below scenarios, which one would you report to the FDA's MedWatch website?

    A. A patient provides you with a forged prescription
    B. An unusual or dangerous side effect has been reported by a patient
    C. The patient wants an early refill
    D. The doctor's prescription has very dangerous medication on it

88. A pharmacy technician can utilize the computer to perform all of the following activities except:

    A. Verify the correctness of a prescription
    B. Place bills to insurance companies
    C. Request a refill from any doctor's office
    D. Request prior authorization from a doctor's office

89. A patient informs you they have developed an allergy to a specific medication. What is your next step?

    A. Give them an EpiPen
    B. Tell the pharmacist about the patient's allergy
    C. Nothing, as the doctor just won't prescribe the medication again
    D. Place the allergy on the patient's profile

90. Which one of the following tasks can be performed by a technician and does not need any intervention from the pharmacist?

    A. Entry of prescription data
    B. Reporting of adverse drug events
    C. DUR
    D. OTC recommendation

Answer Key

Q.	1	2	3	4	5	6	7	8	9	10
A.	B	A	A	A	A	B	B	A	B	C

Q.	11	12	13	14	15	16	17	18	19	20
A.	A	C	C	C	C	A	C	D	C	D

Q.	21	22	23	24	25	26	27	28	29	30
A.	B	D	C	A	B	D	A	C	D	B

Q.	31	32	33	34	35	36	37	38	39	40
A.	C	C	A	A	A	A	D	D	D	C

Q.	41	42	43	44	45	46	47	48	49	50
A.	A	C	B	A	C	B	D	A	C	A

Q.	51	52	53	54	55	56	57	58	59	60
A.	D	A	B	B	A	A	B	A	B	C

Q.	61	62	63	64	65	66	67	68	69	70
A.	C	A	D	B	C	A	C	D	A	D

Q.	71	72	73	74	75	76	77	78	79	80
A.	B	C	B	A	C	A	B	C	A	D

Q.	81	82	83	84	85	86	87	88	89	90
A.	A	C	A	A	D	C	B	A	D	A

Answer Explanations

1.   B: Class II recalls are where the patient may experience temporary adverse effects.

2.   A: You always want to separate your controlled Schedule II drugs from those in the non-controlled Schedule III to V category.

3.   A: The DEA Form 222 lets you order controlled substances.

4.   A: The first two digits need to add up to the last digit.

5.   A: Two to five years is the answer, but this varies based on state laws.

6.   B: When receiving Schedule II medicines, the pharmacist must always verify the date of receipt.

7.   B: The DEA number of the transferring pharmacy must always be noted.

8.   A: The total amount purchased should always be recorded.

9.   B: OSHA ensures employees are always kept safe when performing their duties.

10.   C: All hazardous waste needs to be put in a leakproof container.

11.   A: The more strict law always supersedes.

12.   C: Cost does not result in a recall.

13.   C: CSOS is the acronym.

14.   C: Phenylephrine is not restricted.

15.   C: Toprol is the brand name for metoprolol.

16.   A: Paxil is the brand name for paroxetine, and the dosing is correct.

17. C: Sublingual tablets should be placed under the tongue.

18. D: Enteral means oral medication, so "swallow" is correct.

19. C: A suspension should always be shaken before use to redistribute particles throughout the solution.

20. D: Zoloft's generic name is sertraline.

21. B: Acetaminophen is present in both Percocet and Tylenol.

22. D: This warning is an example of a contraindication, as it can have life-threatening complications.

23. C: A suppository follows a rectal route of administration.

24. A: Any feeling after taking medication can be classified as a side effect.

25. B: Drowsiness is a common side effect of diphenhydramine.

26. D: Overdose of acetaminophen can cause liver failure.

27. A: Roxicet contains acetaminophen.

28. C: Water-based oral solutions are only stable for a maximum of 14 days.

29. D: A nonuniform product is not a sign of incompatibility.

30. B: By dividing 480 mg by 80 mg, you will get how many vials are needed.

31. C: Convert hours to minutes and divide the volume by this.

32. C: Simplify the 1,000 mcg/5 mls to 1 ml and calculate for "x" using 600 mcg as an already known amount.

33. A: Calculate the number of minutes to assist with this answer.

34. A: All drugs should have an expiration date.

35. A: Therapeutic substitution is when a different class of drug is given to the patient to perform the same clinical effects.

36. A: "Dispense as written" means you should only use brand names.

37. D: 68 to 77 degrees Fahrenheit is the standard storage temperature requirement.

38. D: The FDA takes care of all drug safety monitoring.

39. D: Warfarin has a narrow therapeutic index.

40. C: Hive is a true allergy.

41. A: The standard concentration of insulin is 100 units per ml.

42. C: PPIs have the suffix -prazole.

43. B: A tablespoon is equal to 15 ml.

44. A: Convert mls to drops in order to calculate this question.

45. C: Know how to convert from mcg to mg.

46. B: Use the allegations formula to calculate this answer.

47. D: The lot number always needs to be documented.

48. A: One person should be involved in compounding a prescription for the sake of uniformity.

49. C: Simplify to get 1 gram, and you will get the answer.

50. A: Use the allegations formula to calculate this answer

51.   D: PPE should always be donned after you have worked out all the calculations and formulas.

52.   A: Simplify to 1 ml and calculate it as a percentage.

53.   B: A Class A prescription balance is a legal requirement in all pharmacies.

54.   B: A pharmacist is the only one who can verify the prescription during a consultation.

55.   A: This is a simple 'one tablet twice a day for ten days' scenario.

56.   A: Here, you need to know your sig codes.

57.   B: A pharmacist needs to sign off everything you do, especially when reconstituting a drug.

58.   A: An NDC number is 11 digits long.

59.   B: Once you calculate the daily dose, you can divide the total amount of units per vial by that answer.

60.   C: Here, you need to know your sig codes.

61.   C: A lot number is given to all drugs by their manufacturers and can be used in the cases of a recall.

62.   A: If the drug bottle is open, it does not need to be quarantined.

63.   D: This term is known as a medication error.

64.   B: Ensuring that indications are present allows you to match the drugs with the patient's condition.

65.   C: You do not use your asthma pump with the intention of overdosing. You simply want to breathe better.

66. A: The Institute for Safe Medication Practices has authority over all high-alert medications across all healthcare settings.

67. C: High-alert medications have the potential to cause serious considerable harm.

68. D: Hydralazine/hydroxyzine is part of LASA and would benefit from tall man lettering.

69. A: Illegible handwriting is an example of prescriber error.

70. D: This answer sounds the most correct and complete.

71. B: A trailing zero comes after a decimal point.

72. C: This answer sounds the most correct and complete.

73. B: HS can mean both bedtime and half-strength.

74. A: cc can also be confused with units.

75. C: Therapeutic interchange is when an inpatient has their drugs changed.

76. A: The strength of the drug always needs to be present.

77. B: This is simply a missed dose.

78. C: CQI will always aim to improve all pharmacy practices.

79. A: If the patient has side effects, they should be treated immediately. That is always the first step with a medication error.

80. D: ISMP deals with listing all of the inappropriate abbreviations so that pharmacy personnel has a lesser chance of making medication errors.

81. A: Handwashing is the cornerstone of PPE.

82.   C: A barcode system ensures that you are giving the patient the correct medication.

83.   A: Punishing staff members for making medication errors will not help improve the safety of a medication.

84.   A: Always work from dirtiest to cleanest when donning PPE.

85.   D: All members of the pharmacy team can ask a patient whether they would like some counseling by a pharmacist regarding their medications.

86.   C: A pharmacist is the only one allowed to transfer a prescription through an unshared network.

87.   B: MedWatch deals with side effects being present and reported. Especially those that are unusual or dangerous.

88.   A: A pharmacy technician is not allowed to verify the correctness of a prescription.

89.   D: Always make sure that all allergies are on the patient's record for future dispensing purposes.

90.   A: A pharmacy technician can input prescription data without needing any pharmacist intervention.

Chapter Eight: Full-Length Practice Test #3

Questions

1. A script has arrived at your pharmacy, and it says 2 gtt OU BID. What does this mean?

   A. Two drops into both nostrils two times a day
   B. Two drops into both eyes two times a day
   C. Two drops into the left ear three times a day
   D. Two drops into the left eye two times a day

2. What is 25 degrees Celsius in Fahrenheit?

   A. 17 degrees Fahrenheit
   B. 50 degrees Fahrenheit
   C. 77 degrees Fahrenheit
   D. 102 degrees Fahrenheit

3. A boy that is 5'2" and weighs a total of 110 lbs is prescribed a specific drug at a dose of 5 mg/kg. What should his dose be?

   A. 1,300 mg
   B. 1,200 mg

C. 200 mg

D. 250 mg

4. What is CCXL equal to?

A. 2400

B. 275

C. 2040

D. 240

5. A patient is picking up a prescription for Drug F. She is receiving 100 tablets and will be paying a total of $122. How much does each tablet cost?

A. $0.12

B. $1.22

C. $0.012

D. $12.20

6. A Class II recall on a prescription drug will most likely be done by which regulatory agency?

A. FDIC

B. DEA

C. FDA

D. OSHA

7. A cart exchange is a mechanism where non-immediate prescription drugs and equipment are distributed to all patients. The pharmacy is responsible for overseeing all of the orders' filling. In a hospital, when will a cart exchange usually take place?

A. 8 hours

B. 11 hours

C. 24 hours

D. 27 hours

8. What will 2.5 ounces equal if converted into ml?

    A. 75 ml
    B. 28 ml
    C. 5 ml
    D. 750 ml

9. Which schedule, in accordance with the DEA, has the least abuse potential?

    A. Schedule II
    B. Schedule III
    C. Schedule V
    D. Schedule I

10. You receive a script for zolpidem. After how long will the script expire, and how many refills are you able to give?

    A. 12 months and no refills given
    B. 6 months and no refills given
    C. 12 months and 12 refills given
    D. 6 months and 5 refills given

11. You receive a script that says 15 ml PO Q4 PRN. What does it mean?

    A. Take a single teaspoon of medicine as needed every 4 hours
    B. Take 15 ml orally every 4 hours as needed
    C. Take 1 tablespoon orally every 4 hours as needed
    D. Take 2 teaspoons orally every 4 minutes as needed

12. Regarding HIPAA, what is not true?

    A. Assists in ensuring a patient's privacy
    B. Ensures that no fraud and abuse within the healthcare space occurs
    C. Regulates the disclosure of confidential patient information
    D. Assists in decreasing the rate at which errors occur in the pharmacy

13. How can a pharmacy order DEA Schedule III drugs from a wholesaler?

   A. Via a standard invoice
   B. Via a credit memo
   C. Via the use of a DEA Form 222
   D. With guaranteed funds

14. Which class of FDA recall is due to the potential of either death or serious/life-threatening injury?

   A. Class 1
   B. Class 2
   C. Class 3
   D. Class 4

15. A patient weighs 75 lbs. With the adult dosage of the same drug being 400 mg, using Clark's rule, what is the dosage for the patient?

   A. 170 mg
   B. 250 mg
   C. 200 mg
   D. 125 mg

16. Dr. Appelby just received her DEA number, and it is 1988. What will the prefix letters for her DEA registration be?

   A. BD
   B. DA
   C. BA
   D. AD

17. Which needle size will have the largest diameter?

   A. 20 gauge
   B. 18 gauge
   C. 16 gauge
   D. 14 gauge

18. What is rosiglitazone used for?

    A. Anticoagulant
    B. Proton-Pump Inhibitor
    C. Antidiabetic
    D. Statin

19. A _____ will distribute air from a HEPA filter into the work area to establish and maintain an environment that is sterile.

    A. A micron filter fan
    B. A laminar flow hood
    C. A cleaner-room fan
    D. A class 1000 air-fan

20. How many tablespoons are there in 16 oz?

    A. 22
    B. 30
    C. 16
    D. 32

21. For a patient who weighs 218 lbs, what will their weight in Kg be?

    A. 109 Kg
    B. 212 Kg
    C. 329 Kg
    D. 99 Kg

22. For the approval of a new anti-anxiety drug that is very similar to diazepam, which regulatory agency would hold the responsibility?

    A. CIA
    B. OSBRA
    C. FDA
    D. DEA

23. Regarding NaCl (sodium chloride), which concentration would be classified as hypertonic?

    A. 0.900%
    B. 0.009%
    C. 0.090%
    D. 9.000%

24. What type of insulin has the fastest action and will reach the bloodstream in the shortest time?

    A. NPH
    B. Lente
    C. Ultra-Lente
    D. Regular

25. A doctor has a dental practice and has just been given his final DEA number. It is AD380410. What is the final number?

    A. 8
    B. 5
    C. 7
    D. 3

26. What class of drug is benazepril?

    A. Calcium Channel Blocker
    B. ACE Inhibitor
    C. Antifungal
    D. Thiazide Diuretic

27. A prescription that you receive says you need to dispense Restoril 15 mg PRN HS #30. What does this mean?

    A. Take your tablets 30 minutes before you go to bed
    B. Take 1 capsule at bedtime as needed
    C. Take 1 tablet on an empty stomach as needed

D. Take 1 tablet with water as needed

28. A prescription you receive asks for a 12% concentration of a 15 g steroid cream. But, your pharmacy only has 15% and 10% concentrations. How would you make the required product?

    A. 6 g of 15% + 9 g of 10%
    B. 8 g of 15% + 7 g of 10%
    C. 10 g of 15% + 5 g of 10%
    D. 12 g of 15% + 3 g of 10%

29. Your pharmacy operates using a 40% markup along with an additional $1.75 dispensing fee. For 10 sildenafil tablets, the wholesale price is $120.00. What is the retail price?

    A. $191.40
    B. $188.50
    C. $132.25
    D. $170.00

30. Which of the following is a beta blocker?

    A. Amlodipine
    B. Valsartan
    C. Enalapril
    D. Metoprolol

31. A preparation that consists of solid particles which have been dispersed in a liquid vehicle is known as:

    A. Emulsion
    B. Mixture
    C. Suspension
    D. Elixir

32. What is the reference list called that has all approved drug's Therapeutic Equivalence Evaluations published by the FDA?

    A. The Black Book
    B. The Orange Book
    C. The MSDS Book
    D. The Master List

33. What schedule is lorazepam?

    A. DEA Schedule II
    B. DEA Schedule I
    C. DEA Schedule IV
    D. DEA Schedule III

34. The sig for your "right ear" is?

    A. AD
    B. AS
    C. AR
    D. AF

35. In terms of accuracy, which graduated cylinder would be best to measure out 2.75 oz?

    A. 125 ml
    B. 100 ml
    C. 50 ml
    D. 250 ml

36. Mixing drugs together for a particular patient's needs is known as?

    A. Spatulation
    B. Concocting
    C. Compounding
    D. Mixology

37. Which of the following is incorrect?

    A. 555 = DLV
    B. 122 = CXXII
    C. 265 = CCLXV
    D. 159 = CLVIIII

38. If a patient is allergic to alcohol, which preparation should they not use?

    A. Mixture
    B. Syrup
    C. Elixir
    D. Suspension

39. Looking at losartan 25 mg's NDC code, it is 00006-0951-54. What does the 0951 represent?

    A. The product
    B. The dosage form
    C. The manufacturer
    D. The drug's class

40. A patent has been given to a manufacturer for exclusive manufacturing rights of a drug. How many years will the patent last, and when will that time period start?

    A. 10 years from FDA approval
    B. 10 years from the moment it reaches the shelves of pharmacies
    C. 15 years from FDA approval
    D. 20 years from the original filing

41. A patient comes to the pharmacy to pick up his prescription. His employer has prescription drug coverage taken out for him. What is the name of the portion he must pay for his prescription?

    A. Premium
    B. Deductible

C. Member Fees

D. Co-Pay

42. Which of the following temperatures are within room temperature standards?

   A. 89 degrees Fahrenheit
   B. 20 degrees Celsius
   C. 37 degrees Celsius
   D. 65 degrees Celsius

43. A doctor orders an IV infusion that needs to be administered at a rate of 25 ml/hr over a period of 20 hours. What is the total fluid volume that should be given to the ward?

   A. 1.25 L
   B. 500 ml
   C. 1,000 ml
   D. 1.5 L

44. How many teaspoons are there in one ounce?

   A. 5
   B. 3
   C. 6
   D. 9

45. How many tablets will need to be dispensed if the prescription reads: Amoxil 500 mg 1tab PO TID x10D?

   A. 15
   B. 20
   C. 30
   D. 35

46. You receive the same prescription as in Question 45. What condition is most likely being treated?

    A. Urinary Tract Infection
    B. Diabetes
    C. GORD
    D. Hypertension

47. What class of drug is propranolol?

    A. Bronchodilator
    B. ACE Inhibitor
    C. NMDA Receptor Agonist
    D. Beta Blocker

48. Which type of diabetes would be insulin dependent?

    A. Hyperglycemia
    B. Diabetes
    C. Type 1 Diabetes
    D. Type 2 Diabetes

49. In terms of FDA medication recall, which class is the least severe?

    A. Class IV
    B. Class I
    C. Class III
    D. Class II

50. What does the acronym APAP stand for?

    A. Aripiprazole
    B. Aspirin
    C. Acetaminophen
    D. None of the above

51. A tablet that dissolves when placed in between the gum and cheek is most likely which dosage form?

    A. Oral
    B. Buccal
    C. Enteric
    D. Sublingual

52. What should be used to clean a laminar flow hood?

    A. Permanganate
    B. Ammonium Chloride
    C. Sulfuric Iodine
    D. Isopropyl alcohol

53. What does the abbreviation PC mean?

    A. With Meals
    B. After Meals
    C. Before Meals
    D. Potassium Chloride

54. In what circumstances can a generic drug be substituted for a brand name drug?

    A. If the pharmacist says it is okay
    B. If the patient says so
    C. If the pharmacy has the correct drugs to make the switch
    D. Only if the prescriber has approved it

55. A 30 ct bottle of ibuprofen is going for $1.99 in your pharmacy. With the wholesale cost being $1.00, what is the percentage markup?

    A. 49%
    B. 100%
    C. 99%
    D. 75%

56. What protects a drug's brand name from being used without authorization?

    A. Trademark
    B. Agreement
    C. Copyright
    D. Patent

57. Which of the DEA schedules have a very high potential for abuse and are typically not used as medication?

    A. Schedule VI
    B. Schedule V
    C. Schedule III
    D. Schedule I

58. Which type of solution below is characteristically sweetened to make it more palatable?

    A. Mixture
    B. Syrup
    C. Elixir
    D. Suspension

59. Which of the following would not be seen as a violation of HIPAA?

    A. Pharmacy technicians gossip about what medication a patient is using
    B. Not telling the patient and obtaining their permission to disclose their information
    C. A Medicaid patient who is not offered counseling regarding a new drug
    D. Making a patient's records available to a third party

60. Which of the following medications does not need to abide by the PPPA locking cap requirements?

    A. Nitroglycerine
    B. Tolterodine
    C. Clonidine

D. Nitrofurantoin

61. Which one of the drugs below would you not use to treat seizures?

   A. Depakote
   B. Lamictal
   C. Topamax
   D. Tramadol

62. One lb is equal to?

   A. 13 oz
   B. 1 L
   C. 454 grams
   D. 3.2 Kg

63. Oxycontin® is an example of a:

   A. Generic name
   B. Brand name
   C. Colloquial name
   D. Chemical name

64. Regarding the phases of the FDA new drug application, which one involves the use of double-blinded placebo-controlled trials across hundreds or thousands of patients?

   A. Phase IV
   B. Phase II
   C. Phase III
   D. Phase I

65. If water freezes at zero degrees Celsius and boils at 100 degrees Celsius, what will the corresponding temperatures in Fahrenheit be?

   A. 15 degrees Fahrenheit for freeze and 326 degrees Fahrenheit for boil
   B. 32 degrees Fahrenheit for freeze and 212 degrees Fahrenheit for boil

C. 47 degrees Fahrenheit for freeze and 200 degrees Fahrenheit for boil

D. 12 degrees Fahrenheit for freeze and 177 degrees Fahrenheit for boil

66.   The fraction ¾ is the same as:

A. 0.750

B. 0.660

C. 0.0750

D. 7.500

67.   How many milliliters of active ingredient can you expect to find in a 1,500-milliliter solution with a 17.5% strength?

A. 117.5

B. 375.8

C. 500.0

D. 262.5

68.   Metformin is known as which class of drug?

A. Antihypertensive

B. Antidiabetic

C. Antibacterial

D. Antiviral

69.   As a pharmacy technician, you have been asked to take one liter of a 20% solution and repackage it into a one-pint bottle of a 5% solution. Calculate how many bottles you will be able to fill:

A. 8

B. 4

C. 12

D. 5

70.   Which of the following drugs would you use to treat athlete's foot?

A. Sildenafil

B. Fluconazole

C. Valgancyclovir

D. Acetaminophen

71. A drug that ensures that a natural biological action does not occur is also referred to as a:

A. Agonist

B. Inhibitor

C. Antagonist

D. Blocker

72. In terms of bioavailability, which dosage form has the highest one?

A. SL

B. TD

C. PO

D. IV

73. A patient who has diabetes has come to your pharmacy to purchase a glucose meter. Their total comes to $75.94, with the value before tax being $69.99. What percentage of tax has been added to this product?

A. 8.5

B. 9.0

C. 7.5

D. 7.0

74. In accordance with legislation, what is the maximum number of days you can fill a DEA Schedule II drug for?

A. 14 days

B. 28 days

C. 7 days

D. 30 days

75. In a hospital, a rolling cabinet which is used to dispense emergency medication, is also known as a:

    A. Emergency Supply Cart
    B. Red Cart
    C. Crash Cart
    D. Emergency Cart

76. Which drug is not controlled by the DEA?

    A. Valium
    B. Prozac
    C. Tylenol
    D. Phentermine

77. A decision to add new medications onto a hospital's existing formulary is usually made by:

    A. A vote from all the hospital staff
    B. The General Manager of the hospital
    C. Pharmacy and Therapeutics Committee
    D. The physician's board

78. What is the process called when you use a spatula to create an ointment?

    A. Compounding
    B. Spatulation
    C. Mixing
    D. Pharmaceutics

79. What does the acronym PPE stand for?

    A. Personal Protective Equipment
    B. Personal Prevalence Evaluation
    C. Personal and Professional Ethics
    D. Planning Professional Enhancements

80. What class of antibiotic is ceftriaxone?

   A. Fluoroquinolone
   B. Macrolide
   C. Penicillin
   D. Cephalosporin

81. You receive a script with the following instructions for the dispensing of Methylprednisolone 10 mg tablets: 4mg QD x 2D; 30mg QD x 3D; 20mg QD x4D; 10mg QD x 5D. What is the total amount of tablets that should be dispensed?

   A. 50
   B. 35
   C. 40
   D. 30

82. A customer has a prescription for benazepril. Which condition are they most likely treating?

   A. Epilepsy
   B. Staph infection
   C. Hypertension
   D. Ear infection

83. What are the two regulatory bodies that ensure patient safety and quality assurance of medication?

   A. DEA and CDC
   B. DEA and FDA
   C. FDA and CDC
   D. SAHPRA and FDA

84. Your pharmacist has asked you to prepare three liters of a 30% strength solution. However, you only have 8-ounce bottles of 70% strength available. How many bottles will need to be opened to fulfill this request?

    A. 8
    B. 4
    C. 6
    D. 2

85. 600 ml of an IV solution is given over a 5-hour period. What is the flow rate that needs to be utilized?

    A. 2 ml/min
    B. 3 ml/min
    C. 2.4 ml/min
    D. 1.8 ml/min

86. A patient is 138 cm tall and weighs 34 Kg. Using Clark's rule, calculate the dose of this patient, keeping into consideration that the adult dose of the prescribed medication is 400 mg.

    A. 150 mg
    B. 200 mg
    C. 180 mg
    D. 210 mg

87. A patient brings a script that is dated December 17th last year, with the date today being April 21st. Given that the prescription allows five refills, how many fills would the patient receive?

    A. One today with one more refill
    B. None today and no more refills
    C. One today and two more refills
    D. One today and no more refills

88. Which DEA Schedule will your benzodiazepines be classified under?

   A. Schedule III
   B. Schedule IV
   C. Schedule V
   D. Schedule I

89. You receive a prescription that says: Drug X 2 mg/Kg TID. The patient weighs 110 lbs. How many milligrams per day will the patient receive?

   A. 500 mg
   B. 150 mg
   C. 300 mg
   D. 275 mg

90. A senior comes to your pharmacy to purchase a blood pressure monitor. Seeing as they get a discount of 15%, and the monitor is priced at $79.99, what will the final price be, adding on a 5% sales tax?

   A. $71.39
   B. $70.02
   C. $69.54
   D. $72.53

Answer Key

Q.	1	2	3	4	5	6	7	8	9	10
A.	B	C	D	D	B	C	C	A	C	D

Q.	11	12	13	14	15	16	17	18	19	20
A.	C	D	A	A	C	C	D	C	B	D

Q.	21	22	23	24	25	26	27	28	29	30
A.	D	C	D	D	A	B	B	A	C	D

Q.	31	32	33	34	35	36	37	38	39	40
A.	C	B	C	A	B	C	D	C	A	D

Q.	41	42	43	44	45	46	47	48	49	50
A.	D	B	B	C	C	A	D	C	C	C

Q.	51	52	53	54	55	56	57	58	59	60
A.	B	D	B	D	C	A	D	B	C	A

Q.	61	62	63	64	65	66	67	68	69	70
A.	D	C	B	C	B	A	D	C	A	B

Q.	71	72	73	74	75	76	77	78	79	80
A.	C	D	A	D	C	B	C	B	A	D

Q.	81	82	83	84	85	86	87	88	89	90
A.	D	C	B	C	A	B	D	B	C	A

Answers and Explanations

1.   B: The main aspect to realize here is that OU means both eyes.

2.   C: Converting from Celsius to Fahrenheit, you will always add 32.

3.   D: Here, you will need to first convert lbs to Kg, then times it by 5 to get the total mg per weight.

4.   D: C = 100, L is 50. With the X before the L, it means minus 10 = a total of 240.

5.   B: Simply take the total and divide it by 100.

6.   C: The FDA deals with recalls and their classes.

7.   C: A cart exchange will only occur every 24 hours.

8.   A: Here, you need to know how many ounces are equal to one ml.

9.   C: The higher the schedule, the greater its chance for abuse.

10.   D: Zolpidem is Schedule IV, so can have a six-month prescription which includes up to five refills.

11.   C: The main aspect to remember here is that Q4 means every 4 hours.

12.   D: HIPAA focuses on patient safety, instances of fraud, and safeguarding patient information. It does not interfere with error rates in a pharmacy.

13.   A: Only Schedule 2 items need a DEA Form 222. Schedules III to V can use a standard invoice.

14.   A: The lower the class number, the higher the potential for serious injury or death.

15.   C: Here, you will need to understand and use Clark's rule, which is the child's weight in lbs/average adult's weight of 150 lbs, and then multiply that answer with the adult dose.

16. C: Remember, the first letter is the type of job performed, and the second letter is the first letter of the surname.

17. D: The lower the gauge, the larger the diameter of the needle.

18. C: Rosiglitazone is used to treat diabetes.

19. B: Sterile environments use laminar flow hoods to distribute air that has been HEPA filtered.

20. D: Here, you need to know how many tablespoons equal one oz and then times that by 16.

21. D: Go back and refer to how many lbs are in one Kg.

22. C: The FDA deals with approving new medicines.

23. D: NaCl comes in at 0.9%. Seeing as hypertonic means "more concentrated," the correct answer is 9%.

24. D: Regular is the only one that fits the description.

25. A: If incorrect, follow the calculation present in the above chapters.

26. B: Benazepril is an ACE inhibitor used to help treat hypertension.

27. B: Here, the key is knowing that HS means at bedtime.

28. A: Here, you want to use the allegation method oc=f calculating to derive the answer.

29. C: By calculating 40% of the total amount and then adding $1.75, you will get the answer.

30. D: Beta blockers usually end with the suffix -olol, making metoprolol the answer.

31.   C: Solid particles in a liquid are a suspension.

32.   B: Anything regarding therapeutic equivalence will be present in the Orange Book.

33.   C: Lorazepam is a DEA Schedule IV drug.

34.   A: Here, you need to know that the "right ear" is AD.

35.   B: You want to use the graduated cylinder that is closest to the amount of liquid in ml. You will therefore need to convert from oz to ml first to get the total volume. The 100 ml cylinder will then be the closest.

36.   C: Custom mixing of medication for a specific patient is known as compounding.

37.   D: You can never have four Is after each other in roman numerals. It will then need to be represented as IV.

38.   C: Elixirs have alcohol in them.

39.   A: The middle numbers always refer to the product in question.

40.   40 - D: A patent will always last for 20 years, and that time period will always start from the moment the papers have been handed to the FDA for approval.

41.   D: This answer is also known as a co-payment.

42.   B: Room temperature is from 20 to 25 degrees Celsius. Add 32 to teach these values to get the amount in Fahrenheit.

43.   B: Here, it is a simple calculation of multiplying 25 ml by 20 hours.

44.   C: Here, you need to know the conversion between teaspoons and ounces.

45.   C: TID stands for three times per day. This means that if you are taking one

tablet three times per day for 10 days, you will need a total of 30 tablets.

46. A: UTIs are typically treated with penicillin.

47. D: Remember, the suffix -olol is categorical for a beta blocker.

48. C: Patients with Type I diabetes need insulin to survive as their bodies do not make it at all.

49. C: Although the greater the number, the less severe the recall, you will need to know that Class IV does not exist.

50. C: APAP stands for acetaminophen.

51. B: Buccal is between the cheek and gum.

52. D: Isopropyl alcohol is the only stable compound that can be used to clean laminar flow hoods.

53. B: Here, you need to know that PC means "after meals."

54. D: The only way you can switch from a generic name to a brand name is if the prescriber has provided permission to do so.

55. C: If you add 99% of the wholesale cost to itself, you will get the mentioned retail price.

56. A: A patent will ensure that no other manufacturers can create your drug.

57. D: The only DEA Schedule that is not used as a medication is Schedule I.

58. B: Syrups contain flavorings that help with making the medication more palatable.

59. C: HIPAA does not interfere with the counseling you provide to your patients.

60. A: Nitroglycerine is classified as an "emergency medication," which means it does not need a PPPA locking cap.

61. D: Tramadol is used to treat severe pain.

62. C: You need to know what one pound equates to.

63. B: The trademark sign gives it away that this is a Brand Name.

64. C: Phase II typically involves hundreds or thousands of individuals.

65. B: Converting from Celsius to Fahrenheit, you will always add 32.

66. A: This is a simple conversion that can be reviewed in the above chapters.

67. D: Here, you know that 17.5% means 17.5 ml in 100 ml. You then convert the 1.5 L into ml, remove a factor of 100 from each side, and then you are left with 15 multiplied by 17.5, which is the answer.

68. C: Anything regarding therapeutic equivalence will be present in the Orange Book.

69. A: You need to know how many mls are in a pint to do the percentage strength conversions effectively.

70. B: Athlete's foot is typically a fungal infection that will be treated by an antifungal like fluconazole.

71. C: Antagonists ensure that no biological effects occur.

72. D: Maximum bioavailability of 100% is only through the IV route.

73. A: Here, you need to find out the difference between the two amounts and calculate it as a percentage of the total amount.

74. D: Any Schedule II drug can be filled for a period that does not surpass 30 days.

75.   C: A crash cart always has a rolling cabinet for ease of access.

76.   B: Prozac is fluoxetine, one of the few drugs that are not controlled by the DEA.

77.   C: Only the pharmacy and therapeutics committee can make changes to a hospital's formulary.

78.   B: Spatulation is the process whereby a spatula is used to create a mixture or ointment.

79.   A: PPE stands for Personal Protective Equipment.

80.   D: Ceftriaxone is a part of the cephalosporin class of antibacterial antibiotics.

81.   D: Here, it is essential to know that QD means "once daily."

82.   C: Benazepril has the suffix -pril, which is usually associated with ACE inhibitors. These are used to treat hypertension.

83.   B: The FDA and DEA are regulatory bodies that ensure patient safety and quality assurance.

84.   C: Here, you will need to convert your ounces to milliliters, as well as your liters to milliliters, to solve effectively.

85.   A: Here, you need to convert your hours to minutes and then divide 600 ml by that number to get the answer.

86.   B: Here, you will need to understand and use Clark's rule, which is the child's weight in lbs/average adult's weight of 150 lbs, and then multiply that answer with the adult dose.

87.   D: The patient has already used 4/5 of his refills, so after obtaining today still he will be left with zero refills.

88.   B: Benzodiazepines are DEA Schedule IV.

89.   C: Here, you need to convert lbs to Kg and then multiply it by the total dose per day to get the amount of mg the patient will receive.

90.   A: The easiest way to approach this is by first removing 15% of the total price, then calculating 5% and adding it to the discounted price.

Chapter Nine: Bonus: Top 200 Drugs

In order for you to be completely competent as a pharmacy technician, it is advised that you have some recognition of the most common drugs that are present on the market. Luckily for you, we have made the perfect list! These are the top 200 drugs you should know before you enter your PTCB exam:

Medicine	Active ingredient	Class of drug
Lexapro	Escitalopram	Selective serotonin reuptake inhibitor (SSRI)
Vicodin	Acetaminophen and hydrocodone	Analgesic/antipyretic and opioid
Prinivil and Qbrelis	Lisinopril	Angiotensin-converting enzyme (ACE) inhibitor
Zocor	Simvastatin	Statin
Synthroid	Levothyroxine	Thyroid hormone
Amoxil and Trimox	Amoxicillin	Antibacterial (antibiotic)
Zithromax	Azithromycin	Macrolide antibacterial (antibiotic)
Microzide and Aquazide	Hydrochlorothiazide	Thiazide diuretic
Norvasc	Amlodipine	Calcium channel blocker (CCB)
Xanax	Alprazolam	Benzodiazepine
Glucophage	Metformin	Oral antidiabetic
Lipitor	Atorvastatin	Statin
Prilosec	Omeprazole	Proton-pump inhibitor (PPI)
Cipro and Proquin	Ciprofloxacin	Fluoroquinolone (antibiotic)
Zofran	Ondansetron	Antiemetic
Clozaril	Clozapine	Antipsychotic
Lasix	Furosemide	Loop diuretic
Levitra	Vardenafil	PDE5 inhibitor
Sumycin, Ala-Tet, and Brodspec	Tetracycline	Antibacterial (antibiotic)
Heparin sodium	Heparin	Anticoagulant
Valcyte	Valgancyclovir	Antiviral
Lamictal	Lamotrigine	Anticonvulsant
Diflucan	Fluconazole	Antifungal
Tenormin	Atenolol	Beta blocker
SIngulair	Montelukast	Leukotriene inhibitor
Flonase	Fluticasone propionate	Corticosteroid
Zyloprim	Allopurinol	Antigout
Fosamax	Alendronate	Bisphosphonate
Pepcid	Famotidine	H2 receptor antagonist
Omnicef	Cefdinir	Cephalosporin
Yaz	Ethinyl estradiol and drospirenone	Contraceptive (also known as "birth control")

Medicine	Active ingredient	Class of drug
Apresoline	Hydralazine	Antihypertensive
Cogentin	Benztropine	Antiparkinsonian
Tussionex Pennkinetic	Chlorpheniramine and hydrocodone	Antihistamine and narcotic
Paxil	Paroxetine	Selective serotonin reuptake inhibitor (SSRI)
Ativan	Lorazepam	Benzodiazepine
Pyridium	Phenazopyridine	Analgesic
Plaquenil	Hydroxychloroquine	Antimalarial
Lidoderm	Lidocaine	Local anesthetic
Cataflam	Diclofenac	Non-steroidal anti-inflammatory drug (NSAID)
Rayos and Deltasone	Prednisone	Corticosteroid
Zetia	Ezetimibe	Antihyperlipidemic
Evista	Raloxifene	Estrogen modulator
Dilantin	Phenytoin	Anticonvulsant
Lovaza	Omega-3 fatty acids	Antitryglyceride
Zanaflex	Tizanidine	Muscle relaxant
Hytrin	Terazosin	Alpha-1 receptor blocker
Dyrenium	Triamterene	Potassium-sparing diuretic
Altace	Ramipril	Angiotensin-converting enzyme (ACE) inhibitor
Pravachol	Pravastatin	Statin
Risperdal	Risperidone	Antipsychotic
Lunesta	Eszopiclone	Z-drug/hypnotic
Celebrex	Celecoxib	Cyclooxygenase (COX) inhibitor
Premarin	Conjugated estrogens	Estrogen replacement
Avelox	Moxifloxacin	Fluoroquinolone (antibiotic)
Aricept	Donepezil	Acetylcholinesterase inhibitor
Macrobid and Macrodantin	Nitrofurantoin	Antibacterial
Duragesic (skin patch)	Fentanyl	Opioid narcotic
Imdur	Isosorbide mononitrate	Nitrate
Prozac and Sarafem	Fluoxetine	Selective serotonin reuptake inhibitor (SSRI)

Medicine	Active ingredient	Class of drug
Aristocort	Triamcinolone	Corticosteroid
Suboxone	Buprenorphine and naloxone	Narcotic and opioid blockers
Vyvanse	Lisdexamfetamine	Central nervous system (CNS) stimulant
Pamelor	Nortriptyline	Tricyclic antidepressant (TCA)
HumaLOG	Insulin lispro	Rapid-acting insulin
Depacon and Depakote	Sodium valproate	Anticonvulsant
BetaSept and ChloraPrep	Chlorhexidine	Disinfectant/antiseptic
Bentyl	Dicyclomine	Antispasmodic
Imitrex	Sumatriptan	Antimigraine
Protonix	Pantoprazole	Proton-pump inhibitor (PPI)
Lopressor	Metoprolol	Beta blocker
Robitussin	Dextromethorphan and guaifenesin	Antitussive and expectorant
Valium	Diazepam	Benzodiazepine
Viagra	Sildenafil	PDE5 inhibitor
Bactroban	Mupirocin	Antibacterial (antibiotic)
Januvia	Sitagliptin	Antidiabetic
Reglan	Metoclopramide	Dopamine antagonist
Relafen	Nabumetone	Non-steroidal anti-inflammatory drug (NSAID)
Keflex	Cephalexin	Cephalosporin (antibiotic)
Effexor	Venlafaxine	Serotonin-norepinephrine reuptake inhibitor (SNRI)
Boniva	Ibandronate	Bisphosphonate
Zantac	Ranitidine	H2-receptor antagonist
Ex-Lax and Senna Lax	Senna	Laxative
NovoLog	Insulin Aspart	Rapid-acting insulin
Bayer, Ecotrin, and Bufferin	Aspirin	Antipyretic and analgesic
Lioresal	Baclofen	Muscle relaxant
Flagyl	Metronidazole	Antibacterial (antibiotic) and antiprotozoal (antibiotic)
Keppra	Levetiracetam	Anticonvulsant
Colcrys and Mitigare	Colchicine	Antigout

Medicine	Active ingredient	Class of drug
Zyprexa	Olanzapine	Antipsychotic
Avodart	Dutasteride	5-Alpha reductase inhibitor
Tricor and Antara	Fenofibrate	Fibrate
Cardura	Doxazosin	Alpha-1 blocker
Aleve	Naproxen	Non-steroidal anti-inflammatory drug (NSAID)
Aldactone	Spironolactone	Potassium-sparing diuretic
Namenda	Memantine	NMDA antagonist
Methadose	Methadone	Opioid analgesic
Vasotec and Epaned	Enalapril	Angiotensin-converting enzyme (ACE) inhibitor
Tamiflu	Oseltamivir	Antiviral
Requip	Ropinirole	Antiparkinsonian
PC Pen VK and Pen V	Penicillin	Beta-lactam antibacterial (antibiotic)
Strattera	Atomoxetine	Norepinephrine reuptake inhibitor
Ambien	Zolpidem	Z-drug/hypnotic
Advair	Salmeterol and fluticasone	Bronchodilators
Levaquin	Levofloxacin	Fluoroquinolone (antibiotic)
Tofranil	Imipramine	Tricyclic antidepressant (TCA)
Reclast and Zometa	Zoledronic acid	Bisphosphonate
Glucotrol	Glipizide	Antidiabetic
Constulose	Lactulose	Laxative
Aciphex	Rabeprazole	Proton-pump inhibitor (PPI)
Otrexup	Methotrexate	Disease-modifying anti-rheumatic drug (DMARD)
Cleocin	Clindamycin	Antibacterial (antibiotic)
Tylenol	Acetaminophen	Analgesic and antipyretic
Feosol	Ferrous sulfate	Iron supplement
Relpax	Eletriptan	Antimigraine
Carbacot and Robaxin	Methocarbamol	Muscle relaxant
DiaBeta	Glyburide	Antidiabetic
Celexa	Citalopram	Selective serotonin reuptake inhibitor (SSRI)
Benicar	Hydrochlorothiazide and olmesartan	Thiazide diuretic and angiotensin-II blocker

Medicine	Active ingredient	Class of drug
Coreg	Carvedilol	Beta blocker
Spiriva	Tiotropium	Anticholinergic
Xolair	Omalizumab	Monoclonal antibody
Nitrostat (sublingual)	Nitroglycerin	Nitrate
Eliquis	Apixaban	Anticoagulant
Neurontin	Gabapentin	Anticonvulsant
Enbrel	Etanercept	Disease-modifying anti-rheumatic drug (DMARD)
Herceptin	Trastuzumab	Monoclonal antibody
Atripla	Emtricitabine, tenofovir, and efavirenz	Antiretroviral (ARV)
Xarelto	Rivaroxaban	Anticoagulant
Stalevo 50	Levodopa, carbidopa, and entacapone	Antiparkinsonian
Fioricet	Acetaminophen, butalbital, and caffeine	Analgesic, antipyretic, and barbiturate
Levemir	Insulin detemir	Long-acting insulin
Lovenox	Enoxaparin	Low-molecular-weight heparin (LMWH)
Ritalin and Concerta	Methylphenidate	Central nervous system (CNS) stimulant
Crestor	Rosuvastatin	Statin
Xgeva and Prolia	Denosumab	Monoclonal antibody
Pradaxa	Dabigatran	Anticoagulant
Sensipar	Cinacalcet	Calcimimetic
Vesicare	Solifenacin	Antimuscarinic
Haldol	Haloperidol	Antipsychotic
Ala-Cort	Hydrocortisone	Corticosteroid
HumuLIN	Insulin isophane	Intermediate-acting insulin
Isentress	Raltegravir	Integrase inhibitor
Stelara	Ustekinumab	Monoclonal antibody
Mobic	Meloxicam	Non-steroidal anti-inflammatory drug (NSAID)
Remicade	Infliximab	Monoclonal antibody
Nighttime	Acetaminophen and diphenhydramine	Analgesic/antipyretic and antihistamine
Renvela	Sevelamer	Phosphate binder

Medicine	Active ingredient	Class of drug
Fragmin	Dalteparin	Low-molecular-weight heparin (LMWH)
Zoloft	Sertraline	Selective serotonin reuptake inhibitor (SSRI)
Klonopin	Clonazepam	Benzodiazepine
Avalide	Hydrochlorothiazide and irbesartan	Thiazide diuretic and angiotensin-II blocker
Ceftin	Cefuroxime	Cephalosporin (antibiotic)
Nizoral (topical)	Ketoconazole	Antifungal
Lyrica	Pregabalin	Anticonvulsant
Nexium	Esomeprazole	Proton-pump inhibitor (PPI)
Combivent Respimat	Albuterol and ipratropium	Beta-2 agonist and anticholinergic
Niaspan	Niacin	Vitamin B3
Uroxatral	Alfuzosin	Alpha-1 blocker
Biaxin	Clarithromycin	Macrolide antibacterial (antibiotic)
Zomig	Zolmitriptan	Antimigraine
Invokana	Canagliflozin	SGLT-2 inhibitor and antidiabetic
Saxenda and Victoza	Liraglutide	GLP-1 agonist and antidiabetic
Alimta	Pemetrexed	Anticancer
Lotrisone	Clotrimazole and betamethasone	Antifungal and corticosteroid
Avastin	Bevacizumab	Anticancer
Sovaldi	Sofosbuvir	Hepatitis C drug
Gilenya	Fingolimod	Immunomodulator
Epogen	Epoetin alfa	Human erythropoietin
Seroquel	Quetiapine	Antipsychotic
Amaryl	Glimepiride	Antidiabetic
Percocet	Acetaminophen and oxycodone	Analgesic/antipyretic and opioid
SandIMMUNE and Neoral	Cyclosporin	Immunosuppressant
Lantus	Insulin glargine	Long-acting insulin
Cialis	Tadalafil	PDE5 inhibitor
Elavil and Vanatrip	Amitriptyline	Tricyclic antidepressant (TCA)
Lopid	Gemfibrozil	Fibrate

Medicine	Active ingredient	Class of drug
Flo-Pred	Prednisolone	Corticosteroid
Advil	Ibuprofen	Non-steroidal anti-inflammatory drug (NSAID)
Aceon	Perindopril	Angiotensin-converting enzyme (ACE) inhibitor
Desyrel	Trazodone	Antidepressant
Actos	Pioglitazone	Thiazolidinedione
Proscar	Finasteride	5-Alpha reductase inhibitor
Inbrija, Dopar, and Larodopa	Levodopa	Antiparkinsonian
Actonel	Risedronate	Bisphosphonate
ProAir, Ventolin, and Proventil	Albuterol	Beta-2 agonist
Ultram	Tramadol	Opiate narcotic
Sonata	Zaleplon	Z-drug/hypnotic
Zebeta	Bisoprolol	Beta blocker
Zovirax	Acyclovir	Antiviral
Coumadin	Warfarin	Anticoagulant
Luvox	Fluvoxamine	Selective serotonin reuptake inhibitor (SSRI)
Plavix	Clopidogrel	Antiplatelet
Vibramycin and Adoxa	Doxycycline	Tetracycline antibiotic
Hyzaar	Hydrochlorothiazide and losartan	Thiazide diuretic and angiotensin-II blocker
Kytril and Sancuso	Granisetron	Antiemetic
Restoril	Temazepam	Benzodiazepine
Prevacid	Lansoprazole	Proton-pump inhibitor (PPI)
Augmentin	Amoxicillin and clavulanic acid	Penicillin antibiotic and beta-lactam inhibitor
Mevacor and Altoprev	Lovastatin	Statin

Conclusion

The PTCB exam is passable! Let that statement sink in. You are now equipped to tackle anything that the exam has to throw at you. From understanding all the different elements of medications and then applying them within the context of federal and state regulations, your grasp on the subject matter in these two knowledge domains will already secure you a passing grade!

You then started to become a competent pharmacy technician by understanding what it means to ensure patient safety and quality assurance for the medication they require. Round that off with understanding how to read prescriptions, identify sig codes, and even how to generate credit through returning stock to manufacturers, and you are well equipped to obtain your pharmacy technician qualification.

Use all the content in this book as reference material. If you get stuck, go and reread a chapter or a section of a chapter. There is no shame in going back and solidifying your understanding of important concepts. The depth to which you are able to apply all the concepts in this study guide will determine how good of a pharmacy technician you will become. If you put in the time and study this content, you will be gaining so much more than just a pharmacy technician qualification.

Taking any licensure examination can be very stressful. But, that does not mean that it is impossible, no matter how many people say it is. Follow the study hacks we referred to in this book, ensuring you stay healthy and get enough sleep! Do not let the stress of the exam impact your body's overall functioning. This will only make your body unable to function optimally when you need to take the exam!

You've taken the best steps toward your dream of becoming a pharmacy technician. Use the nuggets in this book to guide you in your decision-making and professional development within the healthcare space. If you find this content useful, head on over to Amazon and give us a 5-star review!

You can do anything that you put your mind to. Study hard, and you will always be able to achieve your dreams. Do not let previous failures dictate the direction your future is to take. You've got this—now go forth and live out your dreams! Good luck!

Printed in the USA
CPSIA information can be obtained
at www.ICGtesting.com
LVHW081412111023
760677LV00017B/15